Cambridge Medical Reviews

Neurobiology and Psychiatry   Volume 1

Cambridge Medical Reviews set out to provide regular volumes of critically selected review material in a growing range of emerging and established disciplines within clinical medicine. They will concentrate particularly on areas where advances in basic biomedical science have a substantial contribution to make to the understanding and treatment of disease.

Rigorous standards of selection and editing ensure a reliable, topical and clinically relevant series of volumes, focused to meet the requirements of clinicians and research workers in each discipline.

Neurobiology and Psychiatry

Editor

Robert Kerwin
Institute of Psychiatry, University of London, London, UK

Advisory editors

David Dawbarn
Department of Medicine, Bristol Royal Infirmary, Bristol, UK

James McCulloch
Wellcome Surgical Institute and Hugh Fraser Neuroscience Laboratories, University of Glasgow, Glasgow, UK

Carol Tamminga
Inpatient Program, Maryland Psychiatric Research Center, Baltimore, Maryland, USA

Cambridge Medical Reviews

Neurobiology and Psychiatry
Volume I

EDITOR

ROBERT KERWIN
Institute of Psychiatry, University of London, London, UK

ADVISORY EDITORS

DAVID DAWBARN
Department of Medicine, Bristol Royal Infirmary, Bristol, UK

JAMES McCULLOCH
Wellcome Surgical Institute and Hugh Fraser Neuroscience Laboratories, University of
Glasgow, Glasgow, UK

CAROL TAMMINGA
Inpatient Program, Maryland Psychiatric Research Center, Baltimore, Maryland, USA

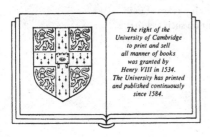

The right of the
University of Cambridge
to print and sell
all manner of books
was granted by
Henry VIII in 1534.
The University has printed
and published continuously
since 1584.

CAMBRIDGE UNIVERSITY PRESS

Cambridge
New York · Port Chester · Melbourne · Sydney

CAMBRIDGE UNIVERSITY PRESS
Cambridge, New York, Melbourne, Madrid, Cape Town,
Singapore, São Paulo, Delhi, Tokyo, Mexico City

Cambridge University Press
The Edinburgh Building, Cambridge CB2 8RU, UK

Published in the United States of America by Cambridge University Press, New York

www.cambridge.org
Information on this title: www.cambridge.org/9780521203494

© Cambridge University Press 1991

First published 1991
First paperback edition 2011

A catalogue record for this publication is available from the British Library

ISBN 978-0-521-39542-7 Hardback
ISBN 978-0-521-20349-4 Paperback

Additional resources for this publication at www.cambridge.org/9780521203494

Contents

	page
Contributors	ix
Editors' preface	xi
Post-mortem neurochemistry of schizophrenia M C ROYSTON and M D C SIMPSON	1
Temporal lobe pathology and schizophrenia G W ROBERTS	15
Frontal lobe, structure, function and connectivity in schizophrenia J M GOLD and D R WEINBERGER	39
Neurotransmitter system abnormalities associated with the neuropathology of Alzheimer's disease D DEWAR	61
Molecular neuropathology of Alzheimer's disease M GOEDERT, M C POTIER and M G SPILLANTINI	95
Neurochemical studies of cortical and subcortical dementias A J CROSS	123
Subcortical dementia – defining a clinical syndrome S FLEMINGER	137
Molecular and cell biology of epilepsy B S MELDRUM and A G CHAPMAN	155
New developments in neuroimaging in schizophrenia L S PILOWSKY and R KERWIN	167
Index	181

Contributors

CHAPMAN, A G, Institute of Psychiatry, De Crespigny Park, Denmark Hill, London SE5 8AF

CROSS, A J, Astra Neuroscience Research Unit, 1 Wakefield Street, London WC1N 1PJ

DEWAR, D, Wellcome Surgical Institute & Hugh Fraser Neuroscience Laboratories, Garscube Estate, Bearsden Road, Glasgow G61 1QH

FLEMINGER, S, Institute of Psychiatry, De Crespigny Park, Denmark Hill, London SE5 8AF

GOEDERT, M, Medical Research Council Laboratory of Molecular Biology, Hills Road, Cambridge CB2 2QH

GOLD, J M, Clinical Brain Disorders Branch, National Institute of Mental Health, NIMH Neuroscience Center at St Elizabeth's, 2700 Martin Luther King Avenue, S E Washington DC 20032, USA

KERWIN, R W, Institute of Psychiatry, De Crespigny Park, Denmark Hill, London SE5 8AF

MELDRUM, B S, Institute of Psychiatry, De Crespigny Park, Denmark Hill, London SE5 8AF

PILOWSKY, L S, Institute of Psychiatry, De Crespigny Park, Denmark Hill, London SE5 8AF

POTIER, M C, Medical Research Council Laboratory of Molecular Biology, Hills Road, Cambridge CB2 2QH

ROBERTS, G W, Department of Anatomy and Cell Biology, St Mary's Hospital Medical School, Norfolk Place, London W2 1PG

ROYSTON, M C, Department of Physiological Sciences, Medical School, Oxford Road, Manchester M13 9PT

SIMPSON, M D C, Department of Physiological Sciences, Medical School, Oxford Road, Manchester M13 9PT

SPILLANTINI, M G, Medical Research Council Laboratory of Molecular Biology, Hills Road, Cambridge CB2 2QH

WEINBERGER, D R, Clinical Brain Disorders Branch, National Institute of Mental Health, NIMH Neuroscience Center at St Elizabeth's, 2700 Martin Luther King Avenue, S E Washington DC 20032, USA

Preface

Neurobiology and Psychiatry Vol I is the first in a series of five volumes within the **Cambridge Medical Reviews** Series.

After several decades of disenchantment with some of the 'biological' aspects of psychiatric research, the past five years have seen tangible progress in the application of basic neurosciences towards understanding the brain mechanisms underlying psychiatric disorders. This is probably because the level of sophistication achieved within the basic sciences is now capable of grappling with the subtle and arcane pathophysiology and biochemistry of human psychiatric disorders. This can now be achieved without resorting to indirect or empirical measures such as animal models or the study of peripheral markers. These volumes will attempt to review, in depth, progress in these areas, concentrating on those conditions and areas where real progress is being made. Volumes I and II will focus primarily on the dementias and schizophrenia, Volume I dealing primarily with neurochemistry, neuropsychology and neuropathology. There still remains much to cover in these areas, and Volume II will also review other fields such as molecular genetics and developmental biology. Topics reviewed in subsequent volumes will depend on areas of future progress, and, in all cases, authors will be chosen from among the most active research workers in biological psychiatry and the neurosciences.

I should like to take the opportunity to thank Professor Shepherd of the Institute of Psychiatry who suggested the project and Richard Barling of CUP for helping to ensure its development and continuity.

Robert Kerwin
Institute of Psychiatry

Post-mortem neurochemistry of schizophrenia

M C ROYSTON AND M D C SIMPSON

Introduction

The notion that schizophrenia has an organic basis has been considered likely for as long as the syndrome has been accepted. In a paper written in 1915 Bleuler[1], responsible for much of the form of our current usage of the term 'schizophrenia' prophetically captured the ideas underpinning contemporary hypotheses of the organic aetiology of schizophrenia:

One must acknowledge that at least the great majority of clinical pictures which are now collected under the name *Dementia praecox* rest on some toxic action or anatomical process which arises independently of psychic influences.

In the ensuing years there have been many studies searching for the abnormal anatomy and toxic substances. These two lines of study examine complementary issues of brain abnormalities apparent at the levels of structural and neurochemical anatomy. In the study of the post-mortem schizophrenic brain there are many important questions which are being addressed by modern neuropathology and neurochemistry. Until recently, there had been little advance in either field but in the last 20 years technical advances and the refinement of research methodologies have produced a new body of evidence which has begun to fit together the pieces which form the jigsaw of schizophrenia.

In neurochemical studies, the initial approach did not focus on the post-mortem brain, but rather on the search for a naturally occurring 'psychomimetic' chemical in the various body fluids of schizophrenic patients. This produced many candidate chemicals and putative markers of aberrant biochemistry all of which have subsequently been dismissed following rigorous scientific enquiry. The endogenous psychotogenic 'pink spot' is a good example of such an endeavour[2].

Post-mortem neurochemistry, in which the substrate of investigation is the

All correspondence to: MC Royston, Department of Physiological Sciences, Medical School, Oxford Road, Manchester M13 9PT, UK.

Cambridge Medical Reviews: Neurobiology and Psychiatry Volume 1
© Cambridge University Press

brain itself, has proved more illuminating. The investigation of the mode of action of those classes of drugs having a beneficial effect in the treatment of schizophrenia has led to the major neurochemical theory of schizophrenia, namely the dopamine theory, which will be considered in detail in this chapter. More broadly than an individual theory, the reversal of at least some of the symptoms of schizophrenia by a drug carries the implication that there is a modifiable chemical abnormality in the brain. This has been a major impetus to the research and development of 'neurochemical' theories of schizophrenia. This approach integrates basic information concerning the chemical and electrical activities, as evidenced by neurotransmitter function, with the higher psychological functioning of the brain, providing a link with the disturbances of thought and perception which characterize the clinical picture of schizophrenia. Over the last 30 years there have been enormous technical advances in the field of analytical biochemistry allowing the chemical identification and quantification of an increasing number of transmitter substances in the central nervous system, many of which have been subsequently implicated in schizophrenia.

The development of complementary techniques for the analysis of neurotransmitter receptors has also been important in stimulating new postmortem neurochemical studies. These methodologies are dependent on the pharmacological principles of ligand binding to specific receptor sites in the tissue studied[3]. By using a ligand labelled with a radioisotope, generally tritium, the sensitive detection technique of radio-assay may be used. Studies may be performed on dissected portions of tissue from post-mortem or more rarely biopsy samples and the pharmacological characteristics of a receptor defined. An image of the distribution of receptors may be made using thin sections of tissue, incubated with a radioligand, and exposed to photographic film. The radiation from the receptor-bound ligand will then produce an image on the film, the intensity of which is in proportion to the tissue concentration of the receptor.

There has also been considerable progress in both neuroimaging and neuropathological studies (reviewed in a later chapter) which provide compelling evidence of a specific structural abnormality of the brain in schizophrenia. Studies of neurochemical pathology can provide complementary 'functional' data to be interpreted in terms of structural pathological findings. Taken together, these lines of evidence support the now prevailing view that schizophrenia is 'no longer a functional psychosis'[4].

Neurotransmitter studies
Three major neurotransmitter systems will be discussed in detail in this review; the dopaminergic system, the neuropeptides and the amino acid neurotransmitters (glutamate and gamma amino butyric acid, GABA). The value of the results from neurochemical studies is critically dependent on the

steps taken to eliminate a number of confounding variables which are inherent in post-mortem studies. These include the effects of agonal state, the deterioration of tissue from the time of death to freezing, the length of storage time, age of subjects, psychiatric diagnosis and selection of control subjects and the drug status of subjects before death with regard to psychoactive medications. Each of these factors may affect adversely the results of the study. For instance, a reduction of GABA content in the amygdala of schizophrenic subjects was reported by Perry et al[5] and by Spokes et al[6] but not by Cross et al[7]. Brain GABA levels were found to rise rapidly after death, thus measurement of the amount of transmitter is an unreliable marker for GABAergic functioning due to dependence on the post-mortem delay. Thus, there have been difficulties in validating findings and the interpretation placed on those findings. More recent studies, paying particular regard to these factors, have produced a degree of convergence in some important areas.

Dopamine

Since the early 1970s, hypotheses implicating abnormalities of central neuro-transmission in the aetiology of schizophrenia have focused in turn on each of the major forebrain monoamine systems. However, no substantial evidence has been produced relating to dysfunction of either the noradrenergic or serotonergic pathways. In contrast, there has been support for overactivity in central dopamine-operated neurones[8]. The 'dopamine hypothesis' has emerged as the primary neurochemical concept, and has been a major influence on biological studies of schizophrenia.

Whilst persuasive, much of the evidence relating to dopamine overactivity in schizophrenia is indirect. This is true of the clinical observations which underpin the hypothesis, the most important of which is the finding that the antipsychotic potency of the neuroleptic drugs is directly related to their affinity as antagonists at the dopamine D2 receptor[9], and the converse observation that drugs which increase central dopamine function such as amphetamine and L-dopa exacerbate the positive symptoms of schizophrenia[10,11]. The inference which has been drawn is that the symptoms of schizophrenia are the consequence of an overactivity of certain dopaminergic pathways[12,13] and that this overactivity is a primary pathophysiological feature of the disease.

Post-mortem examination of the dopamine system has failed to produce unequivocal support for the idea of dopamine dysfunction in schizophrenia. However, for technical reasons the majority of studies have focused on the major target areas of the subcortical dopamine tracts within the basal ganglia, which contain high levels of dopamine, its metabolites and receptors. Whilst a case has been made for an involvement of the basal ganglia in schizophrenia[14], much evidence points to the pathophysiological involvement of the limbic forebrain and cerebral cortex. However, limbic and cortical areas receive a more diffuse dopamine innervation and are less amenable to study. Further technical advances, enabling examination of the mesolimbic and mesocortical dopamine systems at a detailed anatomical level may reveal highly localized and subtle, but critically important, abnormalities.

Dopamine receptor antagonism itself induces adaptive changes at several sites associated with the dopamine neurone. This has been a major difficulty in post-mortem studies of the dopamine system in schizophrenia, since the schizophrenic subjects have almost invariably received neuroleptic medication. The problem then arises of dissociating those effects which are primary to the pathology from those which arise as a result of drug therapy.

Whilst neurotransmitter turnover has been inferred post-mortem from tissue concentrations of transmitters and metabolites, the profound effects of dopamine receptor blockade on dopamine metabolism[15] are a major confounding factor in studies of the brain concentrations of dopamine, its metabolites and associated enzymes. Several studies of this type have been reported, with occasional reports of significant abnormalities within the basal ganglia, but no general consensus. Early reports of increased dopamine concentrations in the caudate nucleus and nucleus accumbens[16,17] were not confirmed in other studies[18], and particularly not in those patients who were drug-free at the time of death[19]. Similarly, there are no marked or consistent changes in the tissue concentration of the major dopamine metabolite homovanillic acid (HVA) in the basal ganglia.

Dopamine metabolism in areas external to the basal ganglia has been less widely examined. However, the report of a unilateral increase in the dopamine concentration of the left amygdala[20] has aroused much interest. Whilst Svendsen et al[21] failed to replicate this finding, a later study by Reynolds[22] confirmed the asymmetric increase in dopamine, with a smaller increase in HVA concentrations. A functional abnormality in amygdalar dopamine would have clear implications, since the amygdala is a key limbic structure, and is a major termination field for the mesolimbic dopamine pathway which has previously been implicated in the production of psychosis and antipsychotic drug action[8]. However, the possibility that this may be a drug-induced effect can not be excluded; Bacopoulos et al[23] described an increase in HVA concentrations in the frontal cortex which was related to previous neuroleptic exposure, and which persisted after long-term exposure to neuroleptic drugs.

Dopamine receptor supersensitivity has repeatedly been proposed to be the substrate for enhanced brain dopamine function. The search for an increased dopamine D2 receptor density in the striatum and nucleus accumbens of schizophrenic subjects[24,25] has been widely confirmed, and was thought to be a primary pathological mechanism, indicating a hypersensitivity of dopaminergic synapses. However, neuroleptic administration to rodents was itself shown to induce an increase in dopamine D2 receptor density[26]. The question of whether drug-naive or drug-withdrawn subjects exhibit dopamine D2 receptor hypersensitivity has been the subject of much research effort. Early studies included reports of either increased[27] or normal[17] striatal dopamine D2 receptor density in unmedicated schizophrenic subjects. More recently, Kornhuber et al[28] in a group of 27 patients demonstrated an increase in D2 density only in those who had received neuroleptics during the 3 months prior to death. However, Seeman et al[29] demonstrated a bimodal distribution of striatal D2 receptor density in 92 schizophrenic subjects, all of whom had received neuroleptic treatment prior to death, concluding that the higher receptor density mode could not be accounted for as an effect of neuroleptic administration alone. The issue remains incompletely resolved, despite the advent of in vivo receptor imaging methods in drug-naive subjects.

Dopamine D1 receptor density has been less widely examined, mainly because of the lack of suitable selective radioligands. Whereas an enhanced activity of the striatal adenylate cyclase associated with the D1 receptor has been reported[30], Carenzi et al[31] found no such abnormality. Several radioligand binding studies of the striatal D1 receptor have failed to demonstrate any significant abnormality[29,32,33], although Hess et al[34] reported a 50% reduction in striatal D1 sites labelled by [^{3}H]-SCH23390. One further possibility which has been considered is that the functional interaction between D1 and D2 receptor activation may be abnormal. Recently, Seeman et al[35] described a direct interaction between the binding of dopamine D1 and D2 selective ligands which was absent in over 50% of the schizophrenic striata examined.

Neuropeptides

As the number of peptide substances identified as candidate neurotransmitters in the central nervous system has increased so the list of potential aetiological factors in schizophrenia has grown. Approximately 25 separate neuropeptides have now been shown to be present within central neurones. Many of these have well-defined and highly specific patterns of distribution within the brain, and clearly serve important roles as central neuroregulators. Fewer than 10 of these substances have been subject to detailed investigation in post-mortem studies of schizophrenic brain.

An interest in the role of particular neuropeptides in schizophrenia has arisen from suggestions that some of these substances may be co-localized in the same neurones as other transmitter substances, and may modulate the effect of the primary transmitters. In particular, there is evidence that CCK is co-localized with tyrosine hydroxylase[36] and may exhibit a functional relationship with dopamine. Neurotensin may be another dopamine co-transmitter. Both of these peptides have been shown to inhibit dopamine agonist-driven behaviours by an action which does not involve direct antagonism of dopamine receptors[37]. Abnormalities of dopamine–neuropeptide interactions are therefore potential pathogenetic mechanisms in schizophrenia. Moreover, distribution studies of certain neuropeptides within the brain have associated them particularly with the limbic cortex, being localized in well-defined neuronal networks. In view of the evidence which implicates limbic system dysfunction in schizophrenia, studies of neuropeptide markers are of great interest, and may provide clues to putative abnormalities of the dopamine system in limbic and cortical areas.

The few studies of peptide transmitters in schizophrenic post-mortem brain which have provided evidence of specific deficits suggest a focus of abnormalities within the temporal lobe. Whilst Kleinman et al[38] and Perry et al[39] reported no abnormalities in CCK concentrations in the entorhinal region, an association between reductions in CCK concentrations in the hippocampus and amygdala and the deficit state or type II symptoms of schizophrenia has been reported[40]. These findings may provide a correlate to neuropathological findings in the temporal lobe, since the deficit state may be particularly associated with ventricular enlargement[41]. Furthermore, CCK receptors have also been shown to be reduced in the hippocampus[42]. However, there is little support for an abnormality of neuropeptide–dopamine interactions in the dopamine termination fields of the basal ganglia. Neurotensin concentrations have been found to be normal[40,43], and, whilst neurotensin receptors were found to be increased in the substantia nigra, this appears to be an effect of neuroleptic medication[44,45].

Amino acids

Glutamate is the putative excitatory neurotransmitter of the cortical pyramidal cells[46] which constitute the cortico-fugal projection to the basal ganglia and limbic system[47], defined pathways within the hippocampus[48,49] together with the intra-cortical and callosal pathways which serve to integrate and interconnect the two cerebral hemispheres[50]. GABA is the major inhibitory transmitter of the cerebral cortex, being associated primarily with short axon interneurons[51,52].

The early interest in glutamate in schizophrenia followed the report of Kim et al[53] of low cerebrosinal fluid glutamate levels in chronic schizophrenic subjects. Although this finding was not replicated by other workers[54], Kim et al[53] put forward a hypothesis in which dysfunction of glutamatergic neurones was held to be of primary importance in schizophrenia. One important tenet of this hypothesis is the functional interrelation of glutamate and dopamine[55,56]. In an early post-mortem brain study by Perry[54] the glutamate content was assayed in 6 brain regions and no differences between control and schizophrenic subjects could be found. In a larger study of 33 schizophrenic and 25 control subjects, Korpi et al[57] examined a wide range of brain areas again finding no significant differences. However, the absolute level of glutamate reflects both the metabolic pool of glutamate and the neuro-transmitter pool which constitutes the smaller of the two. An alternative strategy has been to use the radioligand [³H]-D-aspartate which has a high affinity for the glutamate uptake site and can thus be used as a marker for glutamatergic neurones[58]. In a study of 14 schizophrenic and matched control subjects a variety of limbic structures together with temporal and frontal cortical areas were studied using this radioligand[60]. There was a regionally specific, highly significant bilateral increase in [³H]-D-aspartate binding in the orbito-frontal cortex, the authors suggest this abnormally dense glutamatergic innervation may result from a failure in the normal develop-mental 'pruning' process which re-models the immature callosal/temporal projections to the frontal cortex. The results for the polar temporal cortex showed interesting lateralized effects; although in the overall statistical analysis performed the predicted reduction in [³H]-D-aspartate binding fell short of statistical significance, when the data from each side of the brain were compared for individuals within this area it was found that in 8 of the 14 schizophrenic subjects but only 3 of the 14 control subjects had lower levels of binding on the left.

The post-synaptic glutamatergic receptor system has been well charac-terized. Three receptor sub-types have been identified according to their affinity for exogenous ligands[59]; N-methyl-D-aspartate (NMDA receptor), kainic acid (kainate receptor) and the alpha-amino-3-hydroxy-5-methylisoox-azole-4-propionic acid (AMPA / quisqualate receptor). There is a growing data base of information concerning these receptors in post-mortem investiga-tions of schizophrenia. Studies have focused on temporal structures, includ-ing the limbic components and the frontal cortex.

The results from these studies form a complex picture. In attempting a synthesis it is prudent to note that all the studies were performed on relatively small groups, that by Deakin et al[60] had the largest number of subjects at $n =$ 14. However, an overall picture emerges in which it would seem that there is evidence that in medial temporal structures there is a *reduction* in both pre- and post-synaptic markers for the glutamatergic system whereas there is an *increase* in pre- and post-synaptic markers in medial pre-frontal cortical areas. The significant findings in these studies are summarized in Table 1.

The positive findings in the temporal lobe show an interesting lateraliza-tion, with greater reductions in the left hippocampus[66] and in BA38[60], whereas in the frontal regions, when both hemispheres are considered separately, the increases are bilateral. It is of note that these 2 regions have a significant functional relationship; glutamatergic association fibres from the polar temporal cortex project from the contralateral hemisphere[67].

Investigation of the NMDA receptor complex in schizophrenia is of par-ticular interest following the reports that a single dose of phencyclidine (PCP)

Table 1. *Summary of the significant findings in investigations of the pre- and post-synaptic markers of glutamate neurons*

Ligand	Reference	Area studied	
		Frontal	Temporal
Pre-synaptic glutamate neurones			
[³H]-D-aspartate	60	↑ Ba 11 L + R	↓ Ba 38 L
[³]H-D-aspartate	61	↑ Ba 11 L	–
Post-synaptic glutamate receptors			
NMDA [³H]-MK801	62	–	↑ Putamen
[³H]-MK801	63		↑ Sup Temp gyrus
[³H]-PPP	64		↓ Hippo/ Amygdala
[³H]-TCP	64	↑ Ba 11	
Kainate [³H]-Kainic acid	65	↑ Ba 11	
[³H]-kainic acid	66		↓ CA3/CA4 Hippo. L
[³H]-kainic acid	60	↑ Ba 11 L + R	

can precipitate a schizophrenia-like psychosis in normal subjects. Moreover, it can result in a prolonged exacerbation of illness in previously stabilized patients. Unlike the amphetamine-induced psychosis, that produced by PCP demonstrates both positive and negative / deficit symptoms of schizophrenia. Several lines of evidence now indicate that the highly specific receptor site for the PCP drugs is a site within the ion channel gated by the NMDA-receptor[68]. Preliminary studies attempting the pharmacological manipulation of this system have, so far, not produced evidence of clinical efficacy[69,70]. However, the NMDA receptor forms part of an intricate complex[71] and a clear understanding of the inter-relationship of the individual components will be necessary before the system can be successfully manipulated.

Summary of post-mortem neurochemistry in schizophrenia
It is clear from the preceding review that the neurochemistry of schizophrenia is complex and that a simple 'transmitter deficit' model analogous to the striatal dopamine loss in Parkinson's disease is not likely. Detailed functional

inter-relationships exist between major transmitter systems, e.g. dopamine/glutamate and CCK/dopamine. Any abnormalities must therefore be considered in terms of their effect in a dynamic system. Thus, the findings which underpin the 'dopamine' theory of schizophrenia are being reviewed and integrated with findings from studies of peptide and amino acid neurotransmitters.

Contemporary with the development of neurochemical theories of schizophrenia in the last 20 years has been the renewed interest in the neuro-pathology of schizophrenia. This topic is the subject of review in Chapter 2. Subtle structural abnormalities, focused in temporal limbic components, have been demonstrated and have resulted in 2 important issues. First, do the structural abnormalities result from a degenerative or dysplastic/developmental process. Secondly, the question of abnormal cerebral lateralization of structure in schizophrenia. In considering the significance of these findings and their relationship to disturbed brain *function* in schizophrenia, it is pertinent to integrate neurochemical information.

A developmental disturbance in the normal process of neuronal migration and elimination to produce the final adult cortical arrangement will be reflected in abnormal patterns of receptor distribution. Techniques such as auto-radiography which permit the acquisition of neurochemical data at an anatomical level will be able to study this directly. Moreover, studies of the complex sequential pattern of transmitter/receptor expression during development and their relationship to the developing structure of the brain, when compared to the pattern of structural/neurochemical abnormalities seen in schizophrenia, may provide clues to the timing and nature of the causal insult.

The development of cerebral asymmetries, both structural and neuro-chemical, are a late evolutionary development. Recent neuropathological studies, neurochemical and imaging studies in schizophrenia have suggested that there is an abnormal pattern of cerebral asymmetry in schizophrenia. To address this question, careful methodological design of studies is necessary. Ideally, paired data from the left and right hemisphere of each individual should be considered.

Conclusion
In the last 15 years, studies of post-mortem neurochemistry in schizophrenia have not produced a simple 'neurochemical theory' for schizophrenia. The complex interplay between the structure and function of the brain in the production of the clinical phenomena of schizophrenia is gradually emerging. Future studies which adopt an integrated approach to the study of the neuro-chemical anatomy of schizophrenia may reveal the 'toxic action or anatomical process' which Bleuler predicted.

M C Royston & M D C Simpson

References
(1) Bleuler E. Physisch und psychisch in der pathologie. *Z Neurol Psychisch* 1915; 30:426–75.
(2) Friedhoff JJ, Van Winkel E. Conversion of dopamine to 3,4-dimethoxyphenylacetic acid in schizophrenia patients. *Nature* 1963; 199: 1271–2.
(3) Bennett JP, Yamamura HI. *Neurotransmitter, hormone or drug receptor binding.* HI Yamamura, Ed. New York: Raven Press, 1985: 61–89.
(4) Tyrer P, Mackay A. Schizophrenia: no longer a functional psychosis. *Trends in Neurosc* 1986; 9: 537–8.
(5) Perry TL, Kish SJ, Buchanan J, Hansen S. Gamma-Aminobutyric acid deficiency in brain of schizophrenic patients. *Lancet* 1979; i: 237–9.
(6) Spokes EGS, Garrett NJ, Rossor MN, Iversen LL. Distribution of GABA in post-mortem brain tissue from control, psychotic and Huntington's chorea subjects. J Neurol Sci 1980; 48: 303–13.
(7) Cross AJ, Crow TJ, Owen F. Gamma-aminobutyric acid in the brain in schizophrenia. *Lancet* 1979; i: 560–1.
(8) Stevens JR. An anatomy of schizophrenia? *Arch Gen Psychiat* 1973; 29:177–89.
(9) Creese I, Burt DR, Snyder SH. Dopamine receptor binding predicts clinical and pharmacological potencies of antischizophrenic drugs. *Science* 1976; 192: 481–3.
(10) Angrist B, Sathananthan G, Gershon S. Behavioural effects of L-Dopa in schizophrenic patients. *Psychopharmacologia* 1978; 31: 1–12.
(11) Snyder SH, Banerjee SP, Yamamura HT, Greenberg D. Drugs, Neurotransmitters and schizophrenia. *Science* 1974; 184: 1243–53.
(12) Meltzer HY, Stahl SM. The dopamine hypothesis of schizophrenia: a review. *Schizophrenia Bull* 1976; 2: 19–76.
(13) Seeman P. Brain dopamine receptors. *Pharmacol Rev* 1980; 32: 229–313.
(14) McKenna P. Pathology, phenomenology and the dopamine hypothesis of schizophrenia. *Br J Psychiat* 1987; 151: 288–301.
(15) O'Keefe R, Sharma DF, Vogt M. Effect of drugs used in psychoses on cerebral dopamine metabolism. *Br J Pharmacol* 1970; 38: 287–304.
(16) Bird ED, Spokes EGS, Iversen LL. Increased dopamine concentrations in limbic areas of brain from patients dying with schizophrenia. *Brain* 1979; 102: 347–60.
(17) Mackay AVP, Iversen LL, Rossor M, Spokes E, Bird E, Arregui A, Creese I, Snyder SH. Increased brain dopamine and dopamine receptors in schizophrenia. *Arch Gen Psychiat* 1982; 39: 991–7.
(18) Crow TJ, Owen F, Cross AJ et al. Neurotransmitter enzymes and receptors in post-mortem brain in schizophrenia; evidence that an increase in D2 receptors is associated with the type I syndrome. In: Riederer P, Usdin E, eds. *Transmitter biochemistry of human brain tissue.* London: Macmillan, 1981.
(19) Reynolds GP, Czudek C, Bzowej N, Seeman P. Dopamine receptor asymmetry in schizophrenia. *Lancet* 1987; i: 979.
(20) Reynolds GP. Increased concentrations and lateral asymmetry of amygdala dopamine in schizophrenia. *Nature* 1983; 305: 527–9.
(21) Svendsen CN, Langlais PJ, Benes FM, Bird ED. Monoamine levels in the left and right amygdaloid complex of schizophrenic postmortem brain tissue. In:

Shagass C. et al, eds. *Biological Psychiatry*. Amsterdam: Elsevier, 1986: 1115–17.

(22) Reynolds GP. Post-mortem neurochemical studies in schizophrenia. In: Haefner H, Gattaz WF, Janzarik W, eds. *Search for the causes of schizophrenia*. Heidelberg: Springer, 1987.

(23) Bacopoulos NC, Spokes EG, Bird ED, Roth RH. Antipsychotic drug action in schizophrenic patients: effect on cortical dopamine metabolism after long-term treatment. *Science* 1979; 205: 1405–7.

(24) Owen F, Crow TJ, Poulter M, Cross AJ, Longden A, Riley GJ. Increased dopamine-receptor sensitivity in schizophrenia. *Lancet* 1978; ii: 223–5.

(25) Lee T, Seeman P. Dopamine receptors in normal and schizophrenic human brains. Abstract, *Soc. Neurosci* 1977; 3: 443.

(26) Clow A, Theodorou A, Jenner P, Marsden CD. Changes in rat striatal dopamine turnover and receptor activity during one year's neuroleptic administration. *Eur J Pharmacol* 1980; 63: 135–44.

(27) Lee T, Seeman P. Elevation of brain neuroleptic/dopamine receptors in schizophrenia. *Am J Psychiat* 1980. 137: 191–7.

(28) Kornhuber J, Riederer P, Reynolds GP, Beckmann H, Jellinger K, Gabriel E. [^{3}H]-Spiperone binding sites in post-mortem brains from schizophrenic patients: relationship to neuroleptic drug treatment, abnormal movements, and positive symptoms. *J. Neural Transm* 1989; 75: 1–10.

(29) Seeman P, Bzowej NH, Guan HC, Bergeron C, Reynolds GP, Bird ED, Riederer P, Jellinger K, Tourtellotte WW. Human Brain D1 and D2 dopamine receptors in schizophrenia, Alzheimer's, Parkinson's, and Huntington's diseases. *Neuropsychopharmacology* 1987; 1: 5–15.

(30) Memo M, Kleinman JE, Hanbauer I. Coupling of dopamine D1 recognition sites with adenylate cyclase in nuclei accumbens and caudatus of schizophrenia. *Science* 1983; 221: 1304–7.

(31) Carenzi A, Gillin JG, Guidotti A, Schwartz MA, Trabucchi M, Wyatt RJ. Dopamine-sensitive adenylyl cyclase in human caudate nucleus. A study in control subjects and schizophrenic patients. *Arch Gen Psychiat* 1975; 32: 1056–9.

(32) Pimoule C, Schoemaker H, Reynolds GP, Langer SZ. [^{3}H]-SCH 23390 labeled D1 dopamine receptors are unchanged in schizophrenia and Parkinson's disease. *Eur J Pharmacol* 1985; 114: 235–7.

(33) Cross AJ, Crow TJ, Owen F. [^{3}H]-Flupenthixol binding in post-mortem brains of schizophrenics: evidence for a selective increase in dopamine D2 receptors. *Psychopharmacology* 1981; 74: 122–4.

(34) Hess EJ, Bracha HS, Kleinman JE. Creese I. Dopamine receptor subtype imbalance in schizophrenia. *Life Sci* 1987; 40: 1487–97.

(35) Seeman P, Niznik HY, Guan HC, Booth G, Ulpian C. Link between D1 and D2 dopamine receptors is reduced in schizophrenia and Huntington diseased brain. *Proc Natl Acad Sci USA* 1989; 86: 10156–60.

(36) Hokfelt T, Rehfeld JF, Skirboll L, Ivenmark B, Goldstein M, Markey K. Evidence for co-existence of dopamine and CCK in meso-limbic neurones. *Nature* 1980; 285: 476–8.

(37) Nemeroff CB, Hernandez D, Luttinger D, Kalivas PW et al. Interaction

of neurotensin with brain dopamine systems. *Ann NY Acad Sci* 1982; 400: 330–44.

(38) Kleinman JE, Iadarola M, Govoni S et al. Postmortem measurements of neuro-peptides in human brain. *Psychopharmacol Bull* 1983; 19: 375–7.

(39) Perry RH, Dockray GJ, Dimaline R, Perry EK, Blessed G, Tomlinson BE. Neuropeptides in Alzheimer's disease, depression and schizophrenia. *J Neurol Sci* 1981; 51: 465–72.

(40) Roberts GW, Ferrier IN, Lee Y, Crow TJ, Johnstone EC, Owens DG, Bacarese-Hamilton AJ, McGregor G, O'Shaughnessy D, Polak JM, Bloom SR. Peptides, the limbic lobe and schizophrenia. *Brain Research* 1983; 288: 199–211.

(41) Andreasen NC, Olsen SA, Dennert JW. Smith MR. Ventricular enlargement in schizophrenia: relationship to positive and negative symptoms. *Am J Psychiat* 1982; 139: 297–302.

(42) Farmery SM, Owen F, Poulter M et al. Reduced high affinity cholecystokinin binding in hippocampus and frontal cortex of schizophrenic patients. *Life Sci* 1985; 36: 473–7.

(43) Nemeroff CB, Youngblood WW, Manberg PJ, Prange AJ, Kizer JS. Regional brain concentrations of neuropeptides in Huntington's disease and schizophrenia. *Science* 1983; 221: 972–5.

(45) Uhl GR, Kuhar MJ. Chronic neuroleptic treatment enhances neurotensin receptor binding in human and rat substantia nigra. *Nature* 1984; 309: 350–2.

(46) Fonnum F. Glutamate: a neurotransmitter in mammalian brain. *J Neurochem* 1984; 42: 1–11.

(47) Jones EG. Neurotransmitters in the cerebral cortex. *J Neurosurg* 1986; 65: 135–53.

(48) Storm-Mathisen J. Glutamate in hippocampal pathways. In: DiChiari G, Greisa GL, eds. *Glutamate as a neurotransmitter*. New York: Raven Press, 1981: 43–55.

(49) Peinado JM, Mora F. Glutamic acid as a putative transmitter of the interhemispheric corticocortical connections in the rat. *J Neurochem* 1986; 47: 1598–6030.

(50) DiChiari G, Greisa GL. *Glutamate as a neurotransmitter*. New York: Raven Press, 1981.

(51) Fagg GE, Foster AC. Amino acid neurotransmitters and their pathways in the mammalian central nervous system. *Neuroscience* 1984; 9: 701–27.

(52) Roberts E. Gamma amino butyric acid (GABA): From discovery to visualisation of GABAergic neurons in the vertebrate nervous system. In: Bowery NG, ed. *Actions and interactions of GABA and benzodiazepines*. New York: Raven Press, 1984: 1–37.

(53) Kim JS, Kornhuber HH, Schmid-Burgk W, Holzmuller B. Low cerebrospinal fluid glutamate in schizophrenic patients and a new hypothesis on schizophrenia. *Neurosci Lett* 1980; 20: 379–83.

(54) Perry TL. Normal cerebrospinal fluid and brain glutamate levels do not support the hypothesis of glutaminergic neuronal dysfunction. *Neurosci Lett* 1982; 28: 81–5.

(55) Rowlands GJ, Roberts PJ. Activation of dopamine receptors inhibits calcium-dependent glutamate release from cortico-striatal terminals in vitro. *Eur J Pharmacol* 1980; 62: 241–5.

(56) Sherman AD, Mott J. Direct effect of neuroleptics on glutamate release. *Neuropharmacology* 1984; 23: 1253–6.

(57) Korpi ER, Kleinman JE, Goodman SI, Wyatt RJ. Neurotransmitter amino acids in post-mortem brains of chronic schizophrenic patients. *Psychiat Res* 1987; 22: 291–301.

(58) Cross AJ, Skan WJ, Slater P. The association of [^{3}H]-D-aspartate binding and high affinity glutamate uptake in the human brain. *Neurosci Lett* 1986; 63: 121–4.

(59) Watkins E. Excitatory amino acids – a review. *Ann Rev Pharmacol* 1981; 34: 149–236.

(60) Deakin JFW, Slater P, Simpson MDC, Gilchrist AC, Skan WJ, Royston MC, Reynolds GP, Cross AJ. Frontal cortical and left temporal glutamatergic dysfunction in schizophrenia. *J Neurochem* 1989; 52: 1781–6.

(61) Royston MC, Simpson MDC, Slater P, Deakin JFW. An autoradiographic study in schizophrenia: evidence for an altered laminar distribution of [^{3}H]-D-aspartate binding in orbito frontal cortex. *Schizophrenia Res* 1990; 3: 31–2.

(62) Kornhuber J, Mack-Burkhardt F, Riederer P, Hebenstreit CF, Reynolds GP, Andrews HB, Beckman H. ^{3}H-MK-801 binding sites in postmortem brain regions of schizophrenic patients. *J Neural Transm* 1989; 77: 231–6.

(63) Suga I, Kobayashi T, Ogata H, Toru M. Increased [^{3}H]-MK801 binding sites in post-mortem brains of chronic schizophrenic patients. *Proc 17th Coll Internat Neuro-Psychopharmacol* 1990; S2: 28.

(64) Simpson MDC, Royston MC, Slater P, Deakin JFW. Phencyclidine and sigma receptor abnormalities in schizophrenic post-mortem brain. *Schizophrenia Res* 1990; 3: 32.

(65) Nishikawa T, Takasima M, Toru M. Increased [^{3}H]-kainic acid binding in the pre-frontal cortex in schizophrenia. *Neurosci Lett* 1983; 40: 245–50.

(66) Kerwin RW, Patel S, Meldrum BS, Czudek C, Reynolds GP. Asymmetrical loss of glutamate receptor sub-type in left hippocampus in schizophrenia. *Lancet* 1988; i: 583–4.

(67) Steit P. Glutamate and aspartate as transmitter candidates for systems of the cerebral cortex. In: Jones EG, Peters A, eds. *Cerebral cortex* vol 2. New York: Plenum Press, 1984: 119–43.

(68) Honore T. Excitatory amino acid receptor subtypes and specific antagonists. *Med Res Rev* 1989; 9: 1–23.

(69) Deutsch SI, Weizman A, Goldman ME, Morihisa JM. The sigma receptor: a novel site implicated in psychosis and antipsychotic drug efficacy. *Clin Neuropharmacol* 1988; 11: 105–19.

(70) Tamminga CA, Cascell N, Dixon L, Fakouhi T, Herting RL. Excitatory amino acid pharmacotherapy in schizophrenia. *Clin Neuropharmacol* 1990; 13 (suppl 2): 240.

(71) Zukin SR, Javitt DC. The PCP/NMDA theory of schizophrenia: NMDA receptor pharmacology and clinical implications. *Proc 17th Coll Internat Neuropsychopharmacol* 1990; S2: 31.

Temporal lobe pathology and schizophrenia

G W ROBERTS

Introduction

The 1980s saw the advent of a major paradigm shift in our conception of the aetiology of schizophrenia. The rationale that schizophrenia might best be described as a sane response to an insane world or an inappropriate set of responses to familial strife has been swept away by a flood of careful studies which have documented the existence of structural changes in the brains of schizophrenics. Imaging, morphometry and statistics have rent the veil which shrouded the 'functional psychosis' of schizophrenia revealing the feet (or more accurately brain) of clay. This chapter will chart the course of this scientific voyage and outline how our concept of schizophrenia has changed as a consequence.

In clinical studies of neuropsychiatric disease considerable emphasis is laid on the differential diagnosis of 'functional' psychoses from the dementias – the chronic organic psychoses. In the latter, cognitive and intellectual impairment are known to be related to structural changes in the brain. Throughout this century schizophrenia was (and in some quarters still is) generally viewed as a 'functional' psychosis. This label implies the condition arises from the disorderly activity of neurons with no physical alteration of brain substance.

In spite of the psychological and clinical evidence of brain dysfunction and 'soft' neurological signs in schizophrenia, little progress was made in determining its organic parameters for most of this century and early neuropathological studies were conflicting and controversial[1-6]. Corsellis[2] sorrowfully summed up the lack of direction in the field, concluded that poor experimental design and inadequate technique were largely responsible and advised that only the use of carefully matched samples and quantitative techniques were needed to discern the brain abnormalities underlying psychosis.

The renaissance of research into the neuropathology of schizophrenia dates from the study of Johnstone et al[7] which used computerized tomography to

All correspondence to: Dr GW Roberts, Department of Anatomy and Cell Biology, St Mary's Hospital Medical School, Norfolk Place, London W2 1PG.

Cambridge Medical Reviews: Neurobiology and Psychiatry Volume 1
© Cambridge University Press

quantify the size of the ventricular system in schizophrenics and compared them with a group of age-matched controls. They reported ventricular enlargement in schizophrenics which correlated with the cognitive impairment suffered by the patients but was unrelated to physical treatment (Fig. 1). This study replicated earlier pneumo-encephalographic studies[8,9]. Since the publication of this report, a large number of CT and, more recently, magnetic resonance (MR) studies have also reported ventricular enlargement in schizophrenics[10,11] and supported the idea of an underlying structural abnormality in the brains of many schizophrenic subjects.

The existence of 'hard' evidence of structural abnormalities in the brains of schizophrenic subjects convinced pathologists to re-examine the brain in schizophrenia using the appropriate experimental techniques (i.e. statistical comparison of quantitative data obtained from matched groups). At the present time, several large well-controlled studies have been completed in addition to a host of smaller more detailed investigations. A broad consensus has emerged from this work and, for the first time, it has become possible to outline the parameters of the neuropathology of schizophrenia.

Brain structure in schizophrenia

Brain weight
The total brain weight of an individual is affected by many factors. Height, sex, year of birth and cause of death are just a few of the factors which confuse and complicate the measure[12]. There are few reports of brain weight in schizophrenia and the studies performed in the early decades of the century are open to criticism on both statistical and diagnostic grounds[13]. However, the results produced by three recent studies are reasonably consistent. Each found a significant decrease in brain weight in schizophrenia patients compared with controls after adjusting for such factors as height, weight, sex and year of birth. Brown et al.[13], reported an average reduction of some 100 g or 6% (controls with affective disorder 1468 g, schizophrenics 1366 g *fixed* brain weight), Pakkenberg[14] reported a loss of 109 g or 8% (controls 1314 g, schizophrenics 1205 g *fresh* brain weight) and Bruton[15], in a large prospective study, reported a 30 g loss from each hemisphere (approximately 5% of formalin fixed brain weight). In this latter study a further analysis revealed that brain weight was reduced equally in *both left and right cerebral hemispheres*.

Brain length, area and volume
To date, only two post-mortem studies have examined these parameters. Significant (4%) reductions in brain length (maximum antero-posterior length of the formalin fixed cerebral hemisphere) in both male and female schizophrenics (control male 179 mm, female 173 mm, schizophrenic male

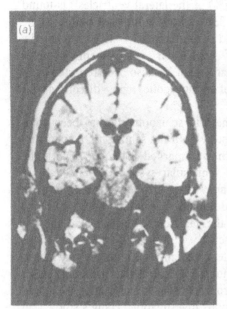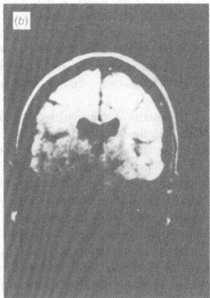

Fig. 1. CT scan in (a) a normal and (b) a schizophrenic male. The enlargement of the ventricular system in the schizophrenic is easily seen.

172 mm and female 164 mm has been reported[13]). A separate analysis indicated that *both* left and right hemispheres were equally reduced in length. Pakkenberg[14] found significant reductions in the volume of the cerebral hemispheres (controls 1046 ml, schizophrenics 959 ml, loss 8%) cerebral cortex (controls 578 ml, schizophrenics 510 ml, loss 12%) and central grey matter (control 48 ml, schizophrenics 45 ml, loss 6%). The volume of the white matter appeared unchanged. Unfortunately, no separate analysis of sex or laterality was made in Pakkenberg's study.

Ventricular system
Several early pneumo-encephalographic studies of the ventricular system in schizophrenia have shown evidence of ventricular dilation[8,9]. However, the ethical problems of such a difficult procedure tempted few to replicate these findings and their significance was gradually forgotten. The advent of computerized tomography (a safer scanning procedure) revitalized clinical interest in the problem and, to date, over 200 computerized tomography (CT) or magnetic resonance imaging (MRI) studies have been carried out and the majority report varying degrees of ventricular enlargement in schizophrenic patients. Post-mortem studies using planimetry have also shown ventricular enlargement. A significant increase in the cross-sectional area of the anterior

17

G W Roberts

horn (+19%) and temporal horn (+97%) of the lateral ventricles[13] is found
and Pakkenberg[14] found an increase of 33% (10 ml) in the total volume of the
ventricular system[14]. Bruton[15] in a blind semi-quantitative study also noted a
significantly increased incidence of ventricular enlargement in their
schizophrenic patients. Ventricular enlargement has also been reported in 13
of 15 affected twins from a series of monozygotic twins discordant for
schizophrenia[16].

The pattern of ventricular enlargement in schizophrenia has been compared with that seen in Alzheimer's disease[17]. In the schizophrenic patients,
the enlargement of the temporal horn was marked (plus 97%) with the
anterior horns and main body of the ventricular system less affected. By
comparison, all regions of the ventricular system were equally enlarged in the
Alzheimer's disease patients. An additional significant finding in the
schizophrenics was a lateralization of the ventricular enlargement, the left
temporal horn being preferentially affected[17].

There is a difference between this latter study and other studies which have
reported ventricular enlargement but not found it to be lateralized. In other
studies, ventricles are assessed from coronal sections rather than in the lateral
view as in this study. In the only previous investigation (Haug's study[8]), in
which measurements were made of ventricular size on a lateral view, the
percentage increase in the component of the ventricle in chronic (by comparison with acute) patients was greatest in the temporal horn and greater on
the left than on the right side of the brain. The fact that these differences are
most apparent from the lateral aspect suggests that the changes in length or
height of the temporal horn are more marked than changes in cross-sectional
area. Indeed, analysis of these parameters[17] showed that changes in temporal
horn height were more significant than changes in length. A structure that
influences the extent of the temporal horn in this dimension is the hippocampus (see below).

The detection of enlarged ventricles using CT and MRI scans are only an
indication of pathology. The resolving power of such techniques is limited and
detailed studies to pin-point specific regions and types of pathological change
require painstaking and reproducible measurements using post-mortem
tissue.

Gyral pattern
Changes in the gyral pattern of the temporal lobe have been described[18].
These findings relate to an autopsy series of 64 schizophrenic patients and a
group of 10 controls. On macroscopic examination they divided the
schizophrenics into two groups. The first with a normal temporal lobe sulco-
gyral pattern ($n = 22$) and the remainder with abnormal sulco-gyral patterns
lobe ($n = 42$). The extent and precise nature of these sulco-gyral pattern
abnormalities were not fully documented. Gyral abnormalities specific to

schizophrenia were not found in a later well-controlled study comparing 52 schizophrenics against 52 controls using either qualitative ratings[15] or a quantitative image analysis technique[19].

Brain regions affected

A quantitative assessment of archival material from patients diagnosed as schizophrenic revealed considerable reductions in the volume of temporal lobe structures (hippocampal formation, amygdala, parahippocampal gyrus) and a moderate reduction of the inner pallidal segment (-20%) in schizophrenic subjects[20]. The outer pallidal segment, caudate, putamen and nucleus accumbens did not show significant volume differences. Significant differences in brain weight were not found (given the sample size – 13 schizophrenics vs 9 controls – this is not surprising). It had been shown previously that volume loss in the amygdala, corpus callosum and internal pallidum in Huntington's chorea and in the substantia nigra in Huntington's chorea and/or Parkinson's disease (both with *no* schizophrenic symptoms) were greater than in patients with schizophrenia[21]. In the light of this, it was concluded[20] that the reduction seen in these structures were not necessarily related to the occurrence of schizophrenic symptoms, and that changes in the hippocampus and medial temporal cortex were specifically related to schizophrenia.

A further planimetric study has also reported similar results[13] comparing 41 schizophrenics and 29 cases of affective disorder. The cases were screened to exclude the presence of senile or vascular change and the findings were controlled for age, sex and year of birth. This study confirmed the presence of ventricular enlargement previously reported in CT scan studies and, in addition, reported that the schizophrenic brains were 6% lighter (see above). The schizophrenic group also had a significantly thinner parahippocampal cortex (by 11%). The thinning of the parahippocampal gyrus correlated significantly with increased area of the temporal horn of the ventricle (Colter, personal communication). No significant differences were noted in the area of the basal ganglia structures, third ventricle, cingulate cortex or the insula opercula cortex. Both of these studies[13,20] reported similar findings of reduced size in schizophrenic brains (although the degree of reduction was less than that found in Alzheimer's disease or Huntington's chorea) and conclude that volume/area reduction is localized rather than general (cf[14]) and, finally, that the temporal lobe, specifically the medial temporal lobe structures (hippocampus and parahippocampal gyrus), are particularly affected.

The link between schizophrenia-like symptoms and the temporal lobe has a long history and, in particular, has been highlighted by Davison and Bagley[22] who documented the association of temporal lobe lesions with schizophrenia-like psychoses occurring in various organic brain disease. In a similar vein, it has been shown that, in patients with temporal lobe epilepsy it is lesions in medial, rather than lateral, temporal lobe structures which are associated with schizophrenia-like psychoses[23]. The post-mortem studies are also supported by a recent MR study[24] which used image analysis to quantify temporal lobe size and the amounts of grey and white matter in schizophrenics. In this study, significant reductions were seen in the amount of temporal lobe grey matter (reduced by 18% right hemisphere, 21% left hemisphere) in schizophrenics which correlated inversely with ventricular enlargement in the same sample. The reductions in temporal lobe grey matter were most pronounced at the level of the amygdala and anterior hippocampus. No differences were seen in the amount of temporal lobe white matter or in the grey or white matter content of the frontal lobes.

Morphology of affected regions

Medial temporal lobe structures particularly the hippocampus have recently been the subject of intensive study. It was reported that the pyramidal cells of the left hippocampal formation display varying degrees of structural disorganization which could be visualized with Golgi impregnation methods and routine histological stains[25]. Neuronal disruption was maximal in the anterior and middle portions of the hippocampus (cf[24]), whereas minimal changes were found posteriorly. The changes particularly affected the interface zones between the entorhinal cortex and the CA1 region and the CA2 and CA3 regions of the hippocampus and were considered to suggest a defective pattern of neuronal migration.

Further data indicating hippocampal dysfunction have been provided. It has been reported that the volumes of the hippocampal formation, pyramidal cell band and the hippocampal segments CA1/CA2, CA3 and CA4 were decreased in the left hemispheres[26]. Pyramidal cell loss was more noticeable in paranoid than in catatonic patients. A trend towards volume reduction was identified in the pre and para subiculum and the perforant path. No significant reductions in volume of the alveus, fimbria and prosubiculum/subiculum were noted. The absolute number of pyramidal cells was reduced in CA1/CA2, CA3 and CA4 zones. The reduction of hippocampal nerve cells was not accompanied by gliosis (as indicated by glial cell counts). The problem with this study (discussed by the authors) is the poor sex-match of the groups (schizophrenics 2 males, 11 females – controls 7 males and 4 females). This is an important point in relation to the author's data showing sex differences in nerve cell densities and absolute cell numbers. Statistical techniques have been used to overcome this difficulty but the finding requires replication. A further study on the same material[27] found reductions in both the area and neuronal content of the entorhinal cortex (no increase in glial cells was observed). Jeste and Lohr[28] have also reported decreased volume of the hippocampus and the pyramidal cell band. The decrease in volume was most marked in the anterior hippocampus of the left side. An interesting preliminary description of morphological changes in the temporal lobe of schizophrenics has also been presented[18] although this study does have methodological handicaps (see[6]). The findings described include alterations to, and cell loss from, the cortical laminae of the ventral insula (claustro-cortex) and in the parahippocampal gyrus. The medial and central portions of the parahippocampal gyrus were most disturbed, and the lateral (transitional) region was less affected. These changes did not extend anterior to the prepiri-form cortex not posterior to the occipital level of the temporal cortex (cf[24,25,28]). The cytoarchitecture of the remaining temporal neocortex was normal. *Both* hemispheres showed changes but they were more conspicuous in the left hemisphere. Of interest was the tendency for patients with marked pathological abnormalities to have an earlier age of onset of psychotic symptoms. The authors suggest that these findings indicate abnormal onto-genetic development of a small part of the entorhinal cortex. In a quantitative study[27] a 20% reduction in neurones was seen in the entorhinal cortex and a preliminary quantitative study of the cyto-architectonics of the pre-alpha cells of the parahippocampal gyrus suggested evidence of putative migration anomalies[29] (Fig. 2).

The prefrontal cortex is also an area of interest following reports of reduced functional activity[30]. A morphometric study of the motor, anterior cingulate and prefrontal cortex in schizophrenia showed a trend toward fewer neurons and cytoarchitectural changes in some cortical layers[31]. Neuronal density was reduced in layer VI of the prefrontal, layer V of the cingulate and layer III of the motor cortex. No differences were found in neuron–glia ratios or neuronal size between schizophrenics and controls. Further analysis showed that in anterior cingulate cortex of schizophrenic patients domains of neurons (par-ticularly in cortical layer II), were smaller in size and separated by a greater distance[32]. Regions of prefrontal and primary motor cortex were not affected similarly. However, no data are given on the gross dimensions of the brains or on the sex matching of the sample (the latter a particularly important issue since sex differences are readily discernible using far less powerful methods of analysis). It should also be noted that these are very subtle changes and it would be interesting to see these techniques applied to the parahippocampal cortex, where cortical thickness is reduced by 11%[13], and neuronal number by 20%[27] and the hippocampus, where a 20% loss of pyramidal neurons may occur[26]. Reductions in volume or cell number have been reported in other brain regions[1-5]. However, changes in other brain regions are neither as marked as those described above nor as consistent.

The process of identifying consistent differences between normal and schizophrenic patients is made more difficult by the findings of neuropatholo-gical surveys which showed that, as a group, the brains of schizophrenic patients shared a high incidence of identifiable pathological changes (e.g. infarcts, vascular disease, Alzheimer-type changes, Parkinson's disease, etc).

21

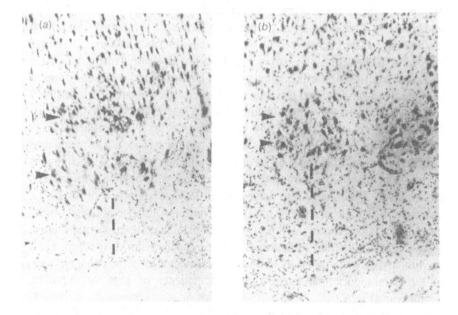

Fig. 2. The cytoarchitecture of the entorhinal cortex (parahippocampal gyrus) is complex. Disorderly arrangement of the layer II (pre-alpha) cells of this region have been reported in schizophrenics. The normal arrangement is shown in (a). An illustration of the disorderly arrangement in schizophrenics is shown (b). Note that the pre-alpha cells will appear not to have developed their typical 'cloud' arrangement (arrow) and have not migrated to their correct position in relation to the pia compared to (a) (dotted line).

Stevens[33] showed identifiable pathology in 50% of cases, Jellinger[3] in 51% and Bruton[15] in 43% (see below for further discussion).

Neuropathological studies of structural changes and clinical symptoms

Searches for a relationship between structural changes and clinical symptoms involving in multiple correlational analyses and as such need to be viewed with a degree of caution. Nevertheless, many of the CT and MRI studies (the techniques of choice in most studies) have similar conclusions in that cognitive impairment (and associated negative symptoms) and measurement of poor pre-morbid and social functioning appear to be best related to the changes in brain structures.

Cognitive impairment (and associated negative symptoms) and measurements of poor pre-morbid and social functioning also appear to be best related to loss of brain weight, decrease in brain length, increased ventricular size and cytoarchitectonic abnormalities[14,15,18]. In general, the greater the structural changes the greater the cognitive impairment and the poorer the pre-morbid function. Cognitive impairment and poor pre-morbid function are associated with early onset of the illness and a poor prognosis[10,11].

Whilst the correlations between measures related to cognitive impairment (negative symptoms or Type II symptoms[34]) and structural changes are discernible, it should be remembered that many of these patients also have delusions and hallucinations (positive or Type I symptoms[34]). Thus, studies in this field are at an early stage and the conclusions concerning the specific clinical correlates of altered morphology should be regarded as preliminary.

The clinical end state of schizophrenia has been viewed as a common endpoint caused by a number of discrete aetiological factors. Various studies have sought to relate measures of structural abnormality (usually ventricular enlargement) to subgroups of schizophrenics defined on the basis of symptomatology or presumed aetiological factors[34-37]. None of these attempts has been entirely convincing. Despite the proposal that ventricular enlargement might be confined to patients with negative symptoms or a history of birth difficulties, ventricular enlargement has been shown in patients with or without positive symptoms, negative symptoms, obstetric complications and with varying degrees of assumed genetic loading[38-41].

It has been proposed that psychiatrists of the future would be able to define subgroups or types of schizophrenia 'according to aetiological principles rather than on the quicksands of symptomatology and course'[42].

At present, there is no consistent evidence that a meaningful sub-grouping of schizophrenics can be made on the basis of the presence or absence of structural change or other aetiological factors. In view of this, and until there is evidence to the contrary, good, scientific practice would lead us to propose that *all* schizophrenics have a degree of structural abnormality and that, neuropathologically, schizophrenia can be viewed as a homogeneous condition. To put it simply, *the symptoms of schizophrenia arise from a type of lesion which differs in degree but not kind*.

Laterality

There is a considerable body of literature describing clinical and psychological observations which suggest that the symptoms of schizophrenia arise from the left or 'dominant' brain hemisphere. In a number of studies, ventricular enlargement has been reported to be more marked in the occipital and temporal horns and to have a degree of selectivity for the left side. For example, Haug[8] found ventricular size to be greater in chronic cases in comparison to acute schizophrenia, and the changes in patients with chronic schizophrenia showed a degree of selectivity to the left temporal horn. An early MRI study found lateral ventricular area to be increased particularly in the posterior (temporal and occipital) coronal sections, and, in those sections in which differences were seen, their significance was greater on the left side[43]. In 25 patients with first episodes of schizophrenia[44], enlargements of the body and occipital and temporal horns were significant on the left but not on the right side, enlargement of the anterior portion of the temporal horn being present only on the left. This finding was consistent with a post-mortem study reporting reduced *temporal lobe area* (with a diagnosis by side-interaction) on the left in patients with schizophrenia by comparison with those with affective disorder[13]. MRI studies have also shown significant reductions in temporal lobe area on the left but not on the right side in chronic schizophrenics[45] and in young patients (mean age of onset 22 years) compared to normal controls[46]. De Lisi[47] reported similar findings in a group of patients with chronic (but not those with acute) schizophrenia.

In an earlier investigation of monozygotic (MZ) twins discordant for schizophrenia[48] a reduction in CT scan density was demonstrated on the left side in the ill twin with significant diagnosis by side interactions particularly in posterior segments. A reduction in scan density might indicate enlargement of csf spaces. Lateralized reductions in volume have also been found in discordant monozygotic twins[16,49]. These studies thus suggest that differences in brain asymmetry can be demonstrated in discordant MZ twins although their precise location remains unclear.

However, whilst some studies have shown changes in some parameters confined to, or more marked on, the left side, it is not in doubt that both hemispheres are affected by structural abnormalities. For example, enlargement of the third ventricle has been reported by a number of workers, and a recent post-mortem study reported that reduction in length and weight was present on both sides of the brain[15].

Aetiology of the structural changes

The original concept of schizophrenia encompassed a degenerative process[50]. This was modified in later years by others to a series of variations of stress-diathesis models and psycho-biological theories. The early CT findings were regarded as evidence for an underlying degenerative process and re-focused attention back to Kraepelin's early ideas. In the early 1980s, schizophrenia was once again viewed as a degenerative process (possibly caused by an acquired pathogen[51]). This view fitted with the correlation between ventricular enlargement and cognitive impairment, a finding to be expected in a neurodegenerative condition.

The report of increased periventricular gliosis[33] was also in accord with a 'low-level of viral infection'. However, the correlation between length of illness and increasing ventricular size seen in other neurodegenerative diseases failed to emerge[10,30,52]. Furthermore, changes of a similar degree were found in patients only weeks or months after the onset of their first episode. Subsequent proposals hypothesized that schizophrenia was of multifactorial aetiology. A number of aetiological factors were proposed of which family history (genetic) and obstetric or perinatal complications (environmental) were regarded as the most prominent[35,53].

Several recent studies have attempted to obtain evidence of the 'smoking gun' which might implicate one of these factors directly. However, the process of identifying aetiological constants in schizophrenics in pathological studies is made more difficult by the findings emerging from neuropathological surveys which showed that, as a group, schizophrenics had a high incidence of identifiable pathological changes (e.g. infarcts, vascular disease, Alzheimer-type changes, Parkinson's disease, etc). Stevens[33] had identifiable pathology in 50% of cases, Jellinger[3] in 51% and Bruton[15] in 43%. In the latter study, the incidence was significantly greater ($P < 0.01$) than the 21% incidence found in age and sex matched controls. The types of pathology found are qualitatively indistinguishable from those seen in age-matched controls, they just occur more frequently[15]. The reason for this 'increased' incidence of pathology is not known although several possibilities have been canvassed[15]. Factors such as lifestyle, drug treatment and, more interestingly, a secondary vulnerability to damage due to underlying structural changes have been raised. However, it is possible that this increase in pathology is merely an artefact due to selection bias since the relative rarity of post-mortem material from schizophrenics encourages a collection at all costs tendency.

Because of the fundamental importance of establishing the aetiology of the disease many neuropathological studies have focused on gathering evidence for the presence of a neurodegenerative process and ascertaining when the structural changes could have occurred. All types of disease process which cause neuronal damage result in a glial reaction marked by the proliferation of glial cells and rises in associated glial proteins (such as glial fibrillary acidic protein GFAP) and enzymes (e.g. monoamine oxidase-B). Establishing a constant pattern of such reactivity in schizophrenic brains would signal the presence of a neurodegenerative process in addition and indicate the location of the damage.

An influential paper[33] reported periventricular gliosis in schizophrenics. However, as noted above, some 50% of these cases had evidence of identifiable pathology. Bruton[15] also noted an increased incidence of gliosis in the schizophrenics. However, detailed analysis showed that this gliosis was significantly associated with the various types of observable pathology present in the brains in the sample. Additional investigations demonstrated that the application of a neuropathological 'sieve' to the total sample (removing cases with identifiable pathology such as senile change but notably excluding gliosis) gave a 'purified' group which still showed reduced brain weight, brain length and increased ventricular size, but this group had no significant gliosis[15]. Since the original quantitative study[54] detailing the lack of gliosis in the brain of schizophrenia, other quantitative studies using similar selection criteria and a variety of methods have reported similar negative results (see

Table 1. *Quantitative assessment of gliosis in schizophrenia*[a]

Method	Ref.	Result
Densitimetry – GFAP stained[b]	54	No gliosis
Cell counts – Nissl stained[b]	26	,,
Cell counts – Nissl stained	31	,,
Densitometry – GFAP stained[b]	55	,,
Assay – monoamine oxidase B	96	,,
Cell counts – Nissl stained[b]	27	,,
Cell counts – GFAP stained	95	,,
Cell counts – GFAP stained	97	,,
Assay – benzodiazepine binding inhibitor peptide[b]	17	,,
Semi-quantitative assessment – Holzer stained[b]	15	,,

[a] Studies using statistical analysis of matched groups.
[b] Sample selected for absence of known pathology (e.g. infarcts, etc).

Table 1). The available pathological evidence indicates that the structural changes in the brains of schizophrenics are not the result of a neurodegenerative process or a destructive lesion. It has been argued that the neuropathological data fit the profile of a disturbance in brain development[55]. Although ideas of aberrant brain development as a cause of schizophrenia have a long history[37], it is only in the later part of the 1980s that such a concept had been firmly rooted in data obtained from direct observation of the neuropathology of the condition.

Abnormal brain development in schizophrenia
Conceiving of schizophrenia as a neurodevelopmental anomaly of the medial temporal lobe gives rise to several predictions[55]. The lesions would be present from birth, preceding the onset of clinical symptoms and may be constant and not progressive. Only a few studies have addressed these questions. Ventricular enlargement has been reported in a 10 year-old diagnosed as schizophrenic[56] and in two teenagers scanned *before* the onset of schizophrenic symptoms[57,58]. There is little or no evidence of progressive structural changes. In the first such study to examine the problem, only 20% of patients were reported showing progressive ventricular enlargement over a 4-year period[9] and recent studies show no evidence of progression in groups of patients scanned over an 8-year interval from 3 to 11 years[59–62], although one recent study has reported a moderate degree of progressive ventricular enlargement[63].

Are these neuropathological data compatible with the intrusion of external environmental events (such as those caused by obstetric complications or infection) on brain development around the time of birth?

Foetal brain tissue does not show an adult glial response until after 6 months[64] and an early destructive lesion might not leave a gliotic trace. However, the type of cytoarchitectonic changes reported in the schizophrenic brain indicate that they originate in the last trimester before birth, a period when an adult-like glial response to injury does occur[64,65]. Birth difficulties can give rise to intraventricular haemorrhages and infarcts that lead to enlarged ventricles and small brains[65,66]. Such pathologies are accompanied by gliosis and perventricular leukomalacia. However, neuropathological studies report no excess gliosis, normal white matter volume and an absence of inflammatory responses[15,54,55] and there is little evidence of traumatic injury[15]. The neuropathological data do not suggest that brain damage due to birth injury or perinatal infection is a major factor in the genesis of the structural abnormalities in schizophrenia. At present there is no direct evidence for the involvement of external environmental events in the genesis of the abnormalities in the brain structure seen in schizophrenics.

The importance of external environmental events in the genesis of brain abnormality is deduced from a number of indirect arguments: (a) the lack of 100% concordance for schizophrenia in monozygotic twins, (b) the excess of winter births in schizophrenics, (c) the increased incidence of birth complications in schizophrenics, and (d) the occurrence of schizophrenic symptoms in various neurological conditions. This evidence has been extensively reviewed[10,22,23,35,37,67].

However, many of these arguments have been criticized. Determination of the percentage of heritability based on monozygotic or dizygotic concordance rates may no longer be valid in general[68] and for schizophrenia in particular it may only represent the lower limit of heritability[69]. This latter study indicates that the genetic risk of developing schizophrenia is the same in descendants of both the ill and the well twin. These data imply that discordance is due to the non-expression or poor penetrance of the genotype rather than the intervention of an environmental event. Accounting for the non-expression of a gene or genes in one of a pair of monozygotic twins is problematic. It has been proposed[68] that, during development at the blastocyst stage, expression of aberrant genes in one part of the cell mass may result in a molecular chimera. The chimera can subsequently undergo fission because one portion of the cell mass fails to recognize the other (what was to be the left side of Harry becomes Fred). The resultant clones (the twin pair) although genetically identical will differ in their expression of the aberrant gene (e.g. monozygotic twins discordant for Duchenne muscular dystrophy[70]). Such a phenomenon could explain some (or all) of the discordance for schizophrenia in monozygotic twins[69].

Re-analysis of the data on excess winter births point to the possibility of an ascertainment artefact in calculating the significance of the phenomenon[71,72]. The significance of birth complications in the pathogenesis of schizophrenia and the direction of causality (i.e. do birth complications cause schizophrenia or does the expression of the schizophrenic genotype cause birth complications?) has been questioned on epidemiological grounds[73]. Although psychotic symptoms indistinguishable from schizophrenia occur during various kinds of neurodegenerative disease[74], notably Alzheimer's disease[75] and temporal lobe epilepsy[23], the incidence of unsuspected organic disease in schizophrenics is only about 5%[76].

Integration of these disparate studies and consideration of them in the light of the neuropathological studies (discussed above) leads this reviewer to the conclusion that the developmental anomaly causing structural changes in the brains of schizophrenics is probably *genetic* in origin in the majority of cases. Environmental factors such as birth complications or other organic disease which might give rise to phenocopies of schizophrenia are 'in all probability' responsible for a small, possibly insignificant, number of cases.

Normal brain development and structural changes in schizophrenia

As outlined above, it has been proposed that a disturbance in the mechanisms of brain development due to a genetic defect could explain the structural changes in the brains of schizophrenics.

The basic sulcogyral pattern of the lower temporal region develops in humans between the seventh and eighth foetal month with the finer relief of the lower convolution occurring in the ninth month and after birth[77]. In contrast, the parahippocampal gyrus is formed approximately at the end of the sixth foetal month, at the same time as the upper temporal region[78]. The first signs of the hippocampal primordium can be observed at 6 weeks in the dorsomedial wall of the embryonic hemisphere and a definite cell lamina of the hippocampus can be detected at seven weeks. The primordium of the entorhinal region is detectable towards the end of the third month[79]. The migratory movements of the human entorhinal region are complete by the end of the sixth month. The formation of the neighbouring temporal iso-cortex and of the hippocampus is finished much later.

Thus there is a differential development both spatially and time wise of the components of the temporal lobe. The human brain develops asymmetrically[77]. The gyral pattern of the temporal lobe develops from the 31st week to term, with the left hemisphere developing 1–2 weeks *later* than the right. The hippocampus develops mainly during the latter half of pregnancy and is approximately 50% of the adult volume at birth. The hippocampi are hemispherically asymmetrical both in size and pattern of growth[78]. The hippocampus forms the medial wall of the temporal horn of the ventricular system. During brain development, ventricular size (as a percentage of brain area), is *reduced*[80]. This is particularly noticeable in the temporal horn whose percentage cross-sectional area is halved between birth and 9 years of age[81]. So the

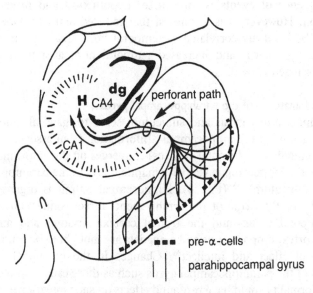

Fig. 3. Anatomical links between the parahippocampal gyrus and the hippocampus. Inputs from many cortical regions synapse in the parahippocampal gyrus. This information is then relayed via the perforant path from the cells of origin in the parahippocampal gyrus to terminate in the hippocampus. Abbreviations: dg, dentate gyrus; H, hippocampus.

volumetric growth of the medial temporal lobe structure causes a compression of the ventricular system and, in particular, the temporal horn.

The development of the parahippocampal gyrus is asymmetric and earlier than the development of the hippocampus. The two structures are functionally connected by the perforant path in (an excitatory glutamatergic projection from the parahippocampal gyrus/entorhinal cortex into the hippocampus; Fig. 3). Loss of, or alteration to, projection systems during *development* can result in aplasia or dystrophy in the target structure (in this case the hippocampus[82]).

Given the parameters governing the pattern of normal brain development, a sequence of events could unfold which provides an explanation for the structural changes seen in the brains of schizophrenics. The genetic mechanism causing the aberration in brain development is effective during the third trimester, it affects both hemispheres and alters the development of the temporal cortex, particularly the parahippocampal gyrus. Since development of the left temporal cortex lags behind the right, any factor which simultaneously affects both will inevitably affect the left more than the right, thus causing asymmetric effects on the (usually symmetrical) growth of the hippocampus. This, in turn, could produce asymmetry of the temporal horn.

G W Roberts

This sequence of events is, of course, hypothetical and needs further investigation. However, it is of interest that reduced temporal lobe volume appears to be inversely correlated to temporal horn area[24] (cf. thinning of parahippocampal gyrus and increased temporal horn area from study of Brown[13] discussed above).

Function and anatomy of the parahippocampal gyrus

The parahippocampal gyrus and subiculum serve to 'gate' all information entering and leaving the hippocampus. Information from association cortex (temporal, cingulate and frontal cortices) converges on the entorhinal cortex and reaches the hippocampus via polysynaptic relays in the parahippocampal gyrus and subiculum[83-85] (Fig. 4). Hippocampal output is organized in a similar fashion. By virtue of the arrangement, direct connections link the medial temporal cortex and the frontal cortex, striatum and amygdala. Temporal cortex, hippocampus and amygdala are thought to be central in the integration of affect and intellect[86]. Changes in the functional ('gating') capabilities of the parahippocampal gyrus such as those caused by a developmental abnormality could have profound effects on such integrative processes and significantly alter the functioning of many other systems (e.g. dorsolateral prefrontal cortex[30,86]). Changes in structure and function caused by the developmental abnormalities will almost inevitably result in alterations in the neurochemical organization of other brain regions. Discussion of the neurochemical changes in the brains of schizophrenics is beyond the scope of the present chapter. There are reports of lateralized changes and these have recently been reviewed[87].

Molecular biology of brain development

How might the genetic defect responsible for brain abnormalities be uncovered? Discrete possibilities about genetic mechanisms are difficult to discern, but recent work in developmental biology may offer significant clues. Two classes of genes have been proposed to be involved in cortical development[88]. One class is thought to regulate the number of radial units (columns) in the cortex. A failure here would reduce the number of columns but the neuronal content *within* each column would remain normal. These defects would be early events in corticogenesis (in humans within 6 weeks of generation), reduced numbers of proliferative radial units are established in the ventricular zone but each unit can produce the normal or genetic number of neurons. Cortex suffering from such defects would have a smaller surface area in spite of normal or enlarged thickness and significant neuronal ectopias (as seen in lissencephaly and pachygyria). This is *not* seen in schizophrenics.

A second class of genes is responsible for the control of neuronal proliferation within radial units. Defects in these genes might cause diminished neuronal production within radial units giving fewer neurons in ontogenetic

30

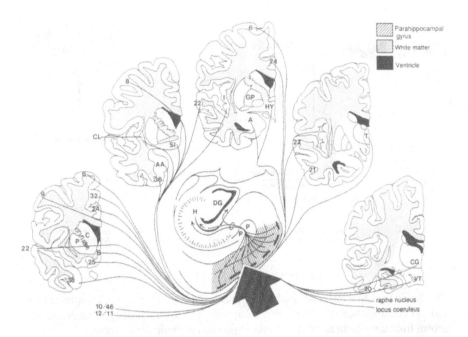

Fig. 4. Projections to the parahippocampal gyrus. The links between various cortical and subcortical areas and the parahippocampal gyrus are shown diagrammatically. The projections shown are those from the same hemisphere, but it should be noted that similar (but smaller) projections from the *opposite* hemisphere are also present. The terminal regions of the projections are topographically organized and often separate projections arise from sub-division of one region (e.g. amygdala). The diagram is a synthesis of data obtained[83-85]. A, amygdala; C, caudate; CL, claustrum; GP, globus pallidus; HY, hypothalamus; P, putamen; S, septum; T, thalamus; AA, anterior amygdala; CG, central grey; DG, dentate gyrus; H, hippocampus; I, insula; PP, perforant path; SI, substantia inominata; VT, ventral tegmentum; 6–46, Brodman areas.

columns and therefore a thinner cortex. Neuronal number in ontogenetic columns could also be affected by programmed cell death or migrational failure. Thinning of the parahippocampal gyrus is seen in schizophrenia and this second class of genes may be worth close study.

Conclusion

The complexity of the genetic regulation of brain development is only just becoming apparent[89,90]. Genes on different chromosomes affect the same cell types, other single genes affect widely different cell types and feedback mechanisms exist between afferents and target cells which determine cell survival and regulate synaptogenesis. Overlaying these mechanisms is the crucial factor in development – that of timing. Widely disparate mechanisms

G W Roberts

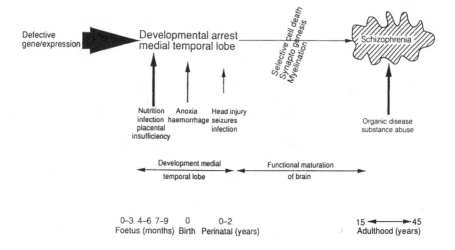

Size of arrow denotes relative importance of factor.

Fig. 5. The relative importance of the various aetiological factors in schizophrenia is shown diagrammatically by the size of the arrows. The natural history of the disease is shown from development through to the expression of clinical symptoms.

(different genes or perturbations in gene expression) operating at the same stage or development produce similar end results. Epidemiologically few cerebral malformations appear to be caused by simple Mendelian inheritance[64]. Studies of common malformations such as an anencephaly, spina bifida and hydrocephalus show a high risk of recurrence in some families. However, analysis of the data suggests an interplay of genetic and environmental factors of which the former is likely to be polygenic[91]. The fine processes which shape brain development could be viewed as an example of a chaotic phenomenon where minor changes in any one of dozens of genes will have unpredictable effects. In such circumstances, arrest or curtailment of cellular migration is more frequent than complete failure, and such phenomena may be more common than previously realized in normal human brains[92].

In schizophrenia, the focus of the abnormality appears to be the parahippocampal cortex with subsequent involvement in other brain areas. The magnitude of the genetic defect and the timing of its expression are probably the factors which determine the extent of the involvement of other brain areas. These developmental anomalies will affect the dynamics of development and cause long-term defects in intellectual function as the brain completes its processes of maturation via mechanisms of programmed cell death, synaptogenesis and myelination[30,93-95] (Fig. 5).

The magnitude of the task of untangling the mechanism(s) which contribute to the schizophrenogenic brain is only now becoming apparent. Many genes could contribute to the structural 'folly' outlined above and none of them may be more important than the others.

Future neuropathological investigations allied to the expansion in our understanding of the genetics of developmental neurobiology augur well for the future and offers a way ahead. Studies will be needed to define the essentials and limits of structural changes in schizophrenia (e.g. cell types affected and altered patterns of neuronal connections) and relate these to the data on factors and mechanisms responsible for the regulation of such phenomena derived from basic studies of brain development. Such progress will inexorably produce the data which eventually enables us to describe the molecular events which, when converted to aberrant brain structure, give rise to the phenomenological condition called schizophrenia.

Acknowledgment
This work was supported by the Theodore and Vada Stanley Foundation.

References
(1) David GB. The pathological anatomy of the schizophrenias. In: Richter D, ed. *Schizophrenia, somatic aspects*. New York: Pergamon, 1957: 93–130.

(2) Corsellis JAN. Psychoses of obscure pathology. In: Blackwood W, Corsellis JAN, eds. *Greenfields neuropathology*. London: Arnold, 1976: 903–15.

(3) Jellinger K. Neuromorphological background of pathochemical studies in the psychoses. In: Beckman H, Reiderer P, eds. *Pathochemical markers in major psychoses*. Heidelberg: Springer, 1985: 1–23.

(4) Roberts GW, Crow TJ. The neuropathology of schizophrenia – a progress report. *Br Med Bull* 1987; 43: 599–615.

(5) Roberts GW. Abnormalities in brain structure in schizophrenia. *Curr Opinion in Psychiat* 1988; 1: 83–9.

(6) Roberts GW, Bruton CJ. Notes from the graveyard: schizophrenia and neuropathology. *Neuropath App Neurobiol* 1990; 16: 3–16.

(7) Johnstone EC, Crow TJ, Frith CD, Husband J, Kreel L. Cerebral ventricular size and cognitive impairment in chronic schizophrenia. *Lancet* 1976; ii: 924–6.

(8) Haug JO. Pneumoencephalographic studies in mental disease. *Acta Psychiatr Scand* 1962; 38: 1–114.

(9) Lemke R. Untersuchungen über die soziale Prognose der Schizophrenia unter besonderer Beruckichtigung des encephalographischen Befundes. *Arch Psychiatr Nervenk* 1935; 104: 89–135.

(10) Crow TJ, Johnstone EC. Schizophrenia: nature of the disease process and its biological correlates. In Plum F, ed. *Handbook of physiology – the nervous system*. Baltimore: Am Physiol Soc 1987; vol 5: 843–69.

(11) Shelton RC, Weinberger DR. X-ray computerised tomography studies of schizophrenia; a review and synthesis. In: *The neurology of schizophrenia*. Nasrallah HA, Weinberger DR, eds. Amsterdam: Elsevier.

(12) Skullerud JR. Variations in the size of the human brain: influence of age, sex,

body length, body mass index, alcoholism, Alzheimer changes and cerebral sclerosis. *Acta Neurol Scand* 1982; 21.

(13) Brown R, Colter N, Corsellis JAN, Crow TJ, Frith CD, Jagoe R, Johnstone EC, Marsh L. Post-mortem evidence of structural brain changes in schizophrenia: differences in brain weight, temporal horn area and parahippo-campal gyrus compared with affective disorder. *Arch Gen Psychiat* 1986; 43: 36–42.

(14) Pakkenberg B. Post-mortem study of chronic schizophrenic brains. *Br J Psychiat* 1987; 151: 744–52.

(15) Bruton CJ, Crow TJ, Frith CD, Johnstone EC, Owens DGC, Roberts GW. Schizophrenia and the brain: a prospective clinico-neuropathology study. *Psych Med* 1990; 20: 285–304.

(16) Suddath RL, Christison GW, Torrey EF, Casanova MF, Weinberger DR. Anatomical abnormalities in the brains of monozygotic twins discordant for schizophrenia. *N Eng J Med* 1990; 322: 789–94.

(17) Crow TJ, Ball J, Bloom SR, Brown R, Bruton CD, Colter N, Frith CD, Johnstone EC, Owens DGC, Roberts GW. Schizophrenia as an anomaly of development of cerebral asymmetry: a post-mortem study and a proposal concerning the genetic basis of the disease. *Arch Gen Psychiat* 1989; 46: 1145–50.

(18) Jakob H, Beckman H. Prenatal developmental disturbances in the limbic allo-cortex in schizophrenics. *J Neural Transmission* 1989; 65: 303–26.

(19) Gentleman S, Williams BJ, Bruton CJ, Vucicevic V, Frith CD, Crow TJ, Roberts GW. Quantitative image analysis in the determination of sulco-gyral pattern variations in the temporal lobe of schizophrenics. *Biol Psychiat*; 29 (suppl 1): 2235.

(20) Bogerts B, Meertz E, Schonfeldt-Bausch R. Basal ganglia and limbic system pathology in schizophrenia: a morphometric study of brain volume and shrinkage. *Arch Gen Psychiat* 1985; 42: 784–91.

(21) Bogerts B. Evidence for structural changes in the limbic system in schizophrenia. *Proc IVth World Congr Biol Psychiat*. Amsterdam: Elsevier/North Holland: 1986.

(22) Davison K, Bagley CR. Schizophrenia-like psychoses associated with organic disorders of the central nervous system – a review of the literature. *Br J Psychiat Spec. Pub. No. 4 Current problems in neuropsychiatry*, Hetherington RN, ed. Kent: Headley Bros Ltd Kent, 1969: 113–84.

(23) Roberts GW, Done DJ, Bruton CJ, Crow TJ. 'A mock up of schizophrenia': schizophrenia-like psychoses and temporal lobe epilepsy. *Biol Psychiat* 1990; 28: 127–43.

(24) Suddath RL, Casanova MF, Goldberg TE, Daniel DG, Kelsoe JR, Weinberger DR. Temporal lobe pathology in schizophrenia: a quantitative magnetic resonance imaging study. *Am J Psychiat* 1989; 146: 464–

(25) Kovelman JA, Schiebel AB. A neurohistological correlate of schizophrenia. *Biol Psychiat* 1984; 191: 1601–21.

(26) Falkai P, Bogerts B. Cell loss in the hippocampus of schizophrenics. *Eur Arch Psychiatr Neurol Sci* 1986; 236: 154–61.

(27) Falkai P, Bogerts B, Rozumek M. Limbic pathology in schizophrenia: the entorhinal region – a morphometric study. *Biol Psychiat* 1988; 24: 515–21.

(28) Jeste D, Lohr JB. Hippocampal pathologic findings in schizophrenia. A morphometric study. *Arch Gen Psychiat* 1989; 46: 1019–24.

(29) Falkai P, Bogerts B, Roberts GW, Crow TJ. Measurement of the alpha-cell-migration in the entorhinal region: a marker for the developmental disturbances in schizophrenia? *Schizophrenia Res* 1988; 1: 157–8.

(30) Weinberger DR. Implications of normal brain development for the pathogenesis of schizophrenia. *Arch Gen Psychiat* 1987; 44: 660–9.

(31) Benes F, Davidson J, Bird ED. Cytoarchitectural studies of the cerebral cortex of schizophrenics. *Arch Gen Psychiat* 1986; 43: 31–5.

(32) Benes FM, Bird ED. An analysis of the arrangement of neurons in the cingulate cortex of schizophrenic patients. *Arch Gen Psychiat* 1987; 44: 608–16.

(33) Stevens J. Neuropathology of schizophrenia. *Arch Gen Psychiat* 1982; 39: 1131–9.

(34) Crow TJ. Molecular pathology of schizophrenia. More than one disease process? *B Med J* 1980; 1: 66–9.

(35) Murray RM, Lewis SW, Reveley AM. Towards an aetiological classification of schizophrenia. *Lancet* 1985; i: 1023–6.

(36) Lewis SW, Murray RM. Obstetric complications, neurodevelopmental deviance and risk of schizophrenics. *J Psychiat Res* 1987; 21: 413–21.

(37) Lewis SW. Congenital risk factors for schizophrenia. *Psych Med* 1989; 19: 5–13.

(38) Farmer A, Jackson R, McGuffin P, Storey P. Cerebral ventricular enlargement in chronic schizophrenia: consistencies and contradictions. *Br J Psychiat* 1987; 150: 324–30.

(39) Nimgaonkar VL, Wessely S, Murray RM. Prevalence of familiality, obstetric complications and structural brain damage in schizophrenic patients. *Br J Psychiat* 1988; 153: 191–7.

(40) McGuffin P, Farmer A, Gottesmann II. Is there really a split in schizophrenia? The genetic evidence. *Br J Psychiat* 1987; 150: 581–92.

(41) Owen MJ, Lewis S, Murray RM. Family history and cerebral ventricular enlargement in schizophrenia. A case control study. *Br J Psychiat* 1989; 154: 629–34.

(42) Murray RM, Forester A. Schizophrenia: is the concept disintegrating? *J Psychopharmacol* 1987; 1: 133–9.

(43) Kelsoe JR, Cadet JL, Pickar D, Weinberger DR. Quantitative neuroanatomy in schizophrenia: a controlled magnetic resonance imaging study. *Arch Gen Psychiat* 1988; 45: 533–41.

(44) Degreef G, Bogerts B, Ashtari M, Lieberman J. Ventricular system morphology in first episode schizophrenia; volumetric study of ventricular subdivisions on MRI. *Schizophrenia Res* 1990; 3: 18.

(45) Johnstone EC, Owens DGC, Crow TJ, Frith CD, Alexandroupoulous K, Bydder G, Colter N. Temporal lobe structure as determined by nuclear magnetic resonance in schizophrenia and bipolar affective disorder. *J Neurol Neurosurg Psychiat* 1989; 52: 736–42.

(46) Rossi P, Stratta P, D'Albenzio L, Tartaro A, Schiazza G, di Michele V, Bolino F, Casacchia M. Reduced temporal lobe area in schizophrenia. *Biol Psychiat* 1990; 27: 61–8.

(47) DeLisi LE, Gupta SM, Hoff A, Shields A, Schwartz J, Halthore S, Anand A.

Brain morphology in first episode cases of schizophrenia. *Schizophrenia Res* 1990; 3: 20.

(48) Reveley MA, Reveley AM, Baldy R. Left hemisphere hypodensity in discordant schizophrenic twins a controlled study. *Arch Gen Psychiat* 1987; 44: 625–32.

(49) Crow TJ. Abnormalities in the brain in schizophrenia. *N Eng J Med* 1990; 323: 545–6.

(50) Kraepelin E. Dementia praecox and paraphrenia. Edinburgh: Livingston. Translated in 1971 by Barclay RM, Robertson GM, New York, RE Krieger.

(51) Crow TJ. Is schizophrenia an infectious disease? *Lancet* 1983; i: 173–5.

(52) Weinberger DR. Computed tomography (CT) findings in schizophrenia: speculations on the meaning of it all. *J Psychiat Res* 1984; 18: 477–90.

(53) Murray RM, Lewis Hon W, Owen MJ, Foerster A. The neurodevelopmental origins of dementia praecox. In: *Schizophrenia – the major issues*, McGuffin P, Bebbington P, eds. London: Heinemann, 1988: 90–107.

(54) Roberts GW, Colter N, Lofthouse R, Bogerts B, Zech N, Crow TJ. Gliosis in schizophrenia. *Biol Psychiat* 1986; 21: 1043–50.

(55) Roberts GW, Colter N, Lofthouse RM, Johnstone EC, Crow TJ. Is there gliosis in schizophrenia? Investigation of the temporal lobe. *Biol Psychiat* 1987; 22: 1459–68.

(56) Woody RC, Bolyard K, Eisenhauer G, Altshuler L. CT scan and MRI findings in a child with schizophrenia. *J Child Neurol* 1987; 2: 105–10.

(57) Weinberger DR. Premorbid neuropathology in schizophrenia. *Lancet* 1988; ii: 959–60.

(58) O'Callaghan E, Larkin C, Remond O, Stack J, Ennis JT, Waddington JL. 'Early onset schizophrenia' after teenage head injury. A case report with magnetic resonance imaging. *Br J Psychiat* 1988; 153: 394–6.

(59) Nasrallah HA, Olson S, McCalley-Whitters M, Chapman S, Jacoby CG. Cerebral ventricular enlargement in schizophrenia: a preliminary follow up study. *Arch Gen Psychiat* 1986; 43: 157–9.

(60) Illowsky BN, Juliano DM, Bigleow LB, Weinberger DR. Stability of CT scan findings in schizophrenia: results of an 8 year follow-up study. *J Neurol, Neurosurg Psychiat* 1988; 51: 209–13.

(61) Vita A, Sacchetti E, Valvassori G, Cazzullo CL. Brain morphology in schizophrenia: a 2–5 year CT scan follow-up study. *Acta Psychiat Scand* 1988; 78: 618–21.

(62) Reveley MA, Chitkara B, Lewis SW. Ventricular and cranial size in schizophrenia: a 4–7 year follow-up. Presentation of IVth Winter Workshop on Schizophrenia, Badgastein, Austria 1988.

(63) Woods BT, Yurgelun-Todd D, Benes FM, Frankenburg FR, Pope HG, McSparren J. Progressive ventricular enlargement in schizophrenia: comparison to bipolar affective disorder and correlation with clinical course. *Biol Psychiat* 1990; 27: 341–52.

(64) Larroche JC. Malformations of the nervous system. In: Adams JM, Corsellis JAN, Duchen LW, eds. *Greenfields Neuropathology*. 4th ed. London: Edward Arnold, 1984: 385.

(65) Volpe JJ. *Neurology of the Newborn*. Philadelphia: WB Saunders, 1987.

(66) Gilles FH, Green BE. Neuropathologic indicators of abnormal development. In: Freeman JM, ed. *Prenatal and perinatal factors associated with brain disorders.* NIH Publication No. 85–1149, 1985: 53–109.

(67) McGuffin P, Murray RM, Reveley AM. Genetic influence on the psychoses. *Brit Med Bull* 1987; 43: 531–6.

(68) Burn J, Corney G. Zygosity determination and types of twinning. In: McGillivray I et al, eds. *Twinning and twins.* London: Wiley, 1988: 7–25.

(69) Gottesman II, Bertelsen A. Confirming unexpressed genotypes for schizophrenia. *Arch Gen Psychiat* 1959; 46: 867–62.

(70) Burn J, Povey S, Boyd Y. Duchenne Muscular Dystrophy in one of monozygotic twin girls. *J Med Genet* 1986; 23; 494–500.

(71) Lewis MS. Age incidence and schizophrenia: Part I. The season of birth controversy. *Schizophrenia Bull* 1989a; 15: 59–73.

(72) Lewis MS. Age incidence and schizophrenia: Part II. Beyond age incidence. *Schizophrenia Bull* 1989b; 15: 75–80.

(73) Goodman R. Are complications of pregnancy and birth causes of schizophrenia? *Dev Med Child Neurol* 1988; 30: 391–406.

(74) Johnstone EC, Cooling NJ, Frith CD, Crow TJ, Owens DGC. Phenomenology of organic and functional psychosis and the overlap between them. *Br J Psychiat* 1988; 153: 770–6.

(75) Drevets WC, Rubin EH. Psychotic symptoms and the longitudinal course of senile dementia of the Alzheimer type. *Biol Psychiat* 25: 39–48.

(76) Johnstone EC, Macmillan JF, Crow TJ. The occurrence of organic disease of possible or probable aetiological significance in a population of 268 cases of first episode schizophrenia. *Psych Med* 1987; 17: 371–9.

(77) Chi Je G, Dooling EC, Gilles FH. Gyral development of human brain. *Ann Neurol* 1977; 1: 86–93.

(78) Kretschman H-J, Kammradt G, Krauthause I, Sauer B, Wingert F. Growth of the hippocampal formation in man. *Biblthca Anat* 1986; 28: 27–52.

(79) Humphrey T. The development of the human hippocampal formation correlated with some aspects of its phylogenetic history. In: Hassler R, Stephan H, eds. *Evolution of the forebrain.* Stuttgart: Thieme, 1966.

(80) Koop M, Rilling G, Herrmann A, Kretschmann H-J. Volumetric development of the fetal telencephalon, cerebral cortex, diencephalon and rhombencephalon including the cerebellum in man. *Biblthca Anat* 1986; 28: 53–78.

(81) Kurihara M, Yamashita S, Miyake S, Yamada M, Iwamoto H. Computed tomography of epileptic children: an investigation of the temporal horn. *No To Hattatsu* 1986; 18: 452–8.

(82) Roberts GW. Brain development and CCK systems in schizophrenia: a working hypothesis. In: Weller M, ed. *International perspectives in schizophrenia research.* London: John Libbey, 1990: 51–69.

(83) Van Hoesen GW. The parahippocampal gyrus. New observations regarding its cortical connections in the monkey. *Trends in Neurosci* 1982; 5: 345–50.

(84) Insausti R, Amaral DG, Cowan WM. The entorhinal cortex of the monkey: II cortical afferents. *J Comp Neurol* 1987a; 264: 356–95.

(85) Insausti R, Amaral DG, Cowan WM. The entorhinal cortex of the monkey: subcortical afferents. *J Comp Neurol* 1987b; 264: 396–408.

(86) Frith CD, Done DJ. Towards a neuropsychology of schizophrenia. *Br J Psychiat* 1988; 153: 437–43.

(87) Reynolds GP. Beyond the dopamine hypothesis: the neurochemical pathology of schizophrenia. *Br J Psychiat* 1989; in press.

(88) Rakic P. Specification of cerebral cortical areas. *Science* 1988; 241: 170–6.

(89) Nowakowski RS. Basic concepts of CNS development. *Child Dev* 1987; 58: 568–95.

(90) McConnell SK. Development and decision making in the mammalian cerebral cortex. *Brain Res Rev* 1988; 13: 1–23.

(91) Kaufman WE, Galaburda AM. Cerebrocortical microdysgenesis in neurologically normal subjects: A histopathologic study. *Neurology* 1989; 39: 238–44.

(92) Carlson M, Earls F, Todd RD. The importance of regressive changes in the development of the nervous system: towards a neurobiological theory of child development. *Psychiat Dev* 1988; 1: 1–22.

(93) Goodman R. Neuronal misconnections and psychiatric disorder. Is there a link? *Br J Psychiat* 1989; 154: 292–329.

(94) Schneider GE. Is it really good to have your brain lesion early? A revision of the 'Kennard Principle'. *Neuropsychologia* 1979; 17: 537–83.

(95) Casanova MF, Saunders R, Stevens J, Kleinman JE. Quantitation of astrocytes in the molecular layer of the dentate gyrus in schizophrenic patients. *Biol Psychiat* 1989; 25: 58A–61A.

(96) Owen F, Crow TJ, Frith CD, Johnson JA, Johnstone EC, Lofthouse R, Owens DGC, Poulter M. Selective decreases of MAO-B activity in post mortem brains from schizophrenic patients with Type II syndrome. *Br J Psychiat* 1987; 151: 514–19.

(97) Stevens CD, Altshuler LL, Bogert B, Falkai P. Quantitative study of gliosis in schizophrenia and Huntington's Chorea. *Biol Psychiat* 1988; 24: 697–700.

Frontal lobe structure, function, and connectivity in schizophrenia

J M GOLD AND D R WEINBERGER

Introduction

In the last 15 years there has been a fundamental reorientation in psychiatric thought about the nature of schizophrenia. The results of recent neuroimaging and post-mortem studies have established that alterations of brain structure are reliably present in patients with this illness[1-3]. This direct evidence of CNS compromise has fostered a reconsideration of the nature of the clinical syndrome. There has been an increased interest in the neuropsychological study of schizophrenia as cognitive impairments have come to be regarded as reflective of underlying brain abnormalities rather than as secondary aspects of psychopathology[4,5]. In keeping with this focus on CNS dysfunction, a number of research groups have highlighted the importance of so-called 'negative' or defect symptoms such as social withdrawal, affective flattening, and motivational deficits[6]. This interest in deficit states stands in sharp contrast to earlier conceptualizations of schizophrenia which emphasized the nature and type of hallucinations, delusions, and formal thought disorder, phenomena which are generally classified as positive symptoms.

While this change in perspective has been dramatic, it is sobering to realize that many, if not most, of the important elements of this reorientation were explicitly present in Kraepelin's original descriptions and conceptualizations of dementia praecox (1919/1971)[7]. He stated, 'We observe a weakening of those emotional activities which permanently form the mainsprings of volition. In connection with this, mental activity and instinct for occupation becomes mute. The result of this part of the morbid process is emotional dullness, failures of mental activities, loss of mastery over volition, of endeavor, and of ability for independent action' (p. 74). From this quote it is clear that Kraepelin considered 'negative' symptoms to be fundamental,

All correspondence to: Dr JM Gold, Clinical Brain Disorders Branch, National Institute of Mental Health, NIMH Neuroscience Center at St Elizabeths, 2700 Martin Luther King Ave. SE, Washington, DC 20032, USA.

defining features of the illness. He also addressed the underlying neuro-pathology of dementia praecox stating

If it should be confirmed that the disease attacks by preference the frontal areas of the brain, the central convolutions and the temporal lobes, this distribution would in certain measure agree with our present views about the site of the psychic mechanisms which are principally injured by the disease. On various grounds it is easy to believe that the frontal cortex, which is specially well developed in man, stands in closer relation to his higher intellectual abilities, and these are the faculties which in our patients invariably suffer profound loss. . . . On the other hand the peculiar speech disorders resembling sensory aphasia and the auditory hallucination, which play such a large part, probably point to the temporal lobe being involved.

(p. 219)

Kraepelin appears to have come to these prescient conclusions primarily based on his understanding of brain behavior relations as well as from several early neuropathological reports.

In this chapter, we will selectively review the results of recent clinical, neuroimaging, neuropsychological and post-mortem studies which support and extend Kraepelin's premonition that schizophrenia is a disease that involves a compromise of the frontal and temporal lobes. The major focus of the chapter is on the role of prefrontal dysfunction, as it is useful from a heuristic point of view to explore which aspects of schizophrenia may be attributed to abnormalities of this brain region. It is important to note at the outset that frontal lobe dysfunction in schizophrenia likely occurs in the context of significant extra-frontal neuropathology. These other structural and neurotransmitter abnormalities may converge in the frontal lobe in an interactive fashion, resulting in behavioral alterations quite similar to those seen following focal frontal lesions. With this interactive model in mind, we will also examine some of the related research literature that suggests that the limbic system, particularly medial temporal lobe structures, may be affected in the illness.

Schizophrenic symptoms and behavioral changes following frontal injury

There is convincing evidence that frontal lobe damage may result in per-sonality, affective, and behavioral changes that are relevant to the study of schizophrenia. The early report of Harlow[8] on the case of Phineaus Gage highlighted his loss of inhibitory controls and balance between intellectual faculties and 'animal propensities'. More recently, Eslinger and Damasio[9] provided a detailed neuropsychological and behavioral analysis of patient EVR who demonstrated marked behavioral changes following the surgical removal of a large orbital meningioma. His social and occupational function-ing declined remarkably, apparently as the result of a significant impairment of his social judgement. His ability to anticipate the likely consequences of his actions and gauge the appropriateness of his behavior were dramatically altered. These changes in social judgement and behavior occurred without any detectable deficits in neuropsychological performance including standard tests of frontal function. Thus, in this patient there is a dissociation of behavioral disinhibition and the more formal cognitive mechanisms that might be expected to play a role in such behaviors. This syndrome of increased behavioral activation and coarsening of personality and judgement, as well as preservation of most intellectual functions, has been related by a number of authors[10,11] to medial orbital lesions.

Of greater interest for the study of schizophrenia is the syndrome of behavioral deactivation which has been noted following more dorsolateral lesions. Luria's[12] richly detailed descriptions of the clinical manifestations of this type of lesion emphasize the patient's global loss of interest in his environment. The patient becomes 'inactive, and inattentive, and does only the simplest and most mechanical actions' (p. 294). There is a loss of complex selective activity which is replaced with 'irrelevant stereotyped acts' (p. 295). Action sequences become simplified, and are often contaminated by per-severations which the patient demonstrates no awareness of. For Luria, this loss of cognitive and behavioral complexity is the result of a weakening of the signal function of inner speech which he considered to be the central form of prefrontal cognitive control. Behavior becomes stimulus-bound, elicited by momentary aspects of the present environment when this form of cognitive control is unavailable. Luria's description of frontal control functions is colored by his emphasis on the role of inner speech in the programming of behavior. Other investigators have emphasized broader notions of control processes[13]. However, the essentials of his description of an overall loss of spontaneity, affective engagement, ability to selectively initiate, sustain, and monitor the results of ongoing behavior have been highlighted by many other researchers as well[11].

The syndrome of behavioral deactivation which follows frontal injury is highly similar to Kraepelin's early description of the volitional deficits seen in many patients with schizophrenia. More recent research on negative symptoms has added an emphasis on the general blunting of emotional responsivity and expressiveness, motor retardation, as well as the apparent impoverishment of ideational activity[14]. This parallel of schizophrenic defect symptoms and those seen following frontal injury is suggestive but is not without complication. The precise definition and measurement of negative symptoms has remained controversial as the effects of drug induced Parkin-sonism, depressed mood, long-term institutionalization, and social with-drawal in response to the press of delusional constructions may be difficult to differentiate on clinical examination[15]. However, it does appear that negative symptoms have some predictive validity in terms of the long-term outcome of illness, intellectual impairment, and possibly structural brain abnormalities, suggesting that these symptoms have an important relationship to the basic pathology of the illness[16].

While behavioral similarities of patients with frontal injuries and the defect symptoms of schizophrenia have been noted by many authors[5,17], frontal dysfunction may play an important role in the behavioral consequences of positive symptoms such as hallucinations or delusions. One striking feature of the illness that is often overlooked is the fact that patients rarely act on their delusions. Most patients do not seek evidence for the truth of their delusions, do not take evasive action to escape their imagined persecutors, and rarely report to the authorities the various plots they have discovered. Thus, many patients appear to be indifferent to their own fantastic ideas to the same extent that they are indifferent to the environment in general. Ironically, the motivational deficits of schizophrenic patients may be beneficial in this limited domain of action.

Luria highlights the role of the frontal lobe in the ability to critically examine one's own behavior, to put an action in a general context of long-term goals and the constraints of the current situation. The loss of this critical faculty would appear to be involved in the maintenance of delusional belief. Many patients have wildly implausible beliefs that are explicitly contradicted by even a superficial consideration of their personal history and knowledge of the everyday world. The possibility that frontal dysfunction is involved in this loss of critical evaluation is supported by reports of confabulation, anosognosia and Capgras syndrome following frontal lesions[11,18,19]. These syndromes all involve a fundamental loss of self-awareness and the ability to monitor one's own behavior.

In the case of these unusual neurologic symptoms a combination of frontal and extra-frontal injury is typically involved. Thus, there may be an interactive effect of basic perceptual or mnestic information processing deficits of extra-frontal origin and abnormalities in self-monitoring that result in these types of complex behaviors. The importance of these symptoms is that they can be seen as being on a continuum with frank psychotic symptoms in terms of the degree of reality distortion, suggesting that the frontal cortex may be involved in the genesis and maintenance of psychosis as part of an interactive system. In a very different research context, this concept is also supported by the work of Pycock et al.[20], who demonstrated that the destruction of prefrontal dopamine terminals in the rat resulted in increases of dopamine metabolites in the striatum and limbic system. Thus the loss of normal frontal inhibition may have dramatic effects in connected downstream dopamine-rich limbic regions. In the Pycock model, a primary frontal lesion has neurochemical consequences that may be relevant to the hypothesis that psychosis involves a hyperdopaminergic state of the limbic system. In a series of recent studies, Jaskiw and Weinberger[21] have extended the Pycock model to show that disconnection of prefrontal regions from limbic sites leads to exaggerated responses to environmental stress and dysregulation of limbic dopamine activity. In the previously mentioned example of Capgras syndrome, it is hypothesized that the frontal lobe fails to monitor the dysfunctional output of another region. While the directionality of these models may differ, in both cases the frontal cortex is implicated in the origins of behaviors that may have relevance for psychosis.

It is important to emphasize that complex persistent behavioral phenomena such as hallucinations, delusions, or amotivational states are unlikely to be the result of a single, specific localizable abnormality in the brain. Psychosis following frontal injury is an infrequent occurrence. Several authors have proposed that the limbic system is a more likely site for the genesis of psychosis[22,23]. The evidence for this view includes the observation that limbic injury is more frequently associated with psychotic symptoms[24] and that unusual psychic 'experiential' phenomenon may result from direct electrical stimulation of the anteromedial temporal lobe[25-27]. The 'psychic experiences' studied with direct electrical stimulation in patients with epilepsy bear some resemblance to positive symptoms seen in schizophrenia. However, there appear to be important differences as well. Psychic experiences are often of visual scenes while auditory hallucinations are more common in schizophrenia. The unusual psychic phenomenon reported following electrical stimulation are generally brief in duration and the patient is aware that an unusual state has occurred. Further, patients typically have normal affective responses to the unusual ideas or percepts that they experience. Thus, there does not appear to be the loss of awareness and affective responsivity following electrical stimulation that is seen typically in schizophrenia. Thus it is likely that neither frontal nor limbic lesions alone provide an adequate model of the positive and negative symptoms of schizophrenia. However, the frontal cortex may be a necessary element in the functional systems that are responsible for both the positive and negative symptoms that are fundamental features of schizophrenia.

Frontal dysfunction and cognitive impairment in schizophrenia

The neuropsychological study of the frontal lobes has been marked by extensive controversy. Many studies have failed to document an effect of frontal damage on a wide range of tests of intelligence, memory, attention, and language. Alternately, there have been frequent reports of difficulties in abstract thinking, response planning and inhibition, shifting of set, and the use of information to monitor and correct ongoing behavioral performance following frontal lobe injury[11]. Several recent theoretical accounts of prefrontal cognitive function emphasize the concept of an 'executive' control capacity that is only called into play in relatively novel situations which require the discovery and application of rules or strategies[13]. Global cognitive impairment would not be expected from a patient with executive dysfunction as it is thought that routine, familiar tasks, the manipulation of overlearned information, and tasks which can be solved in a perceptually straightforward fashion should remain unaffected as they do not require executive processes to come into play. Such a model may explain the seemingly contradictory findings of impaired and preserved performance among frontal injury patients reported in the literature.

Empirically, the Wisconsin Card Sorting Test[28] has been shown to be sensitive to frontal lobe lesions, particularly lesions of the dorsolateral prefrontal cortex[29]. Impairment on this task would be expected based on an executive control model of the frontal cortex as the task requires the abstraction of concepts, the maintenance of a conceptual set in the face of distracting, ambiguous stimuli, and the use of feedback to guide performance. The subject must actively form and test hypotheses as the correct sorting principle is shifted without warning. Thus, the task involves nearly all the cognitive dimensions that have been proposed in the literature as being subserved by the frontal cortex.

In a review of work with non-human primates, Goldman-Rakic[30] has suggested that the frontal cortex is the neural substrate of 'working memory'. Her concept of working memory is colored by the primate experimental paradigms sensitive to frontal lesions, i.e. delayed alternation and delayed response. In each task the monkey must be able to sustain a representation of the immediately preceding stimulus configuration over a delay interval in order to plan and correctly execute their next response. This ability to 'hold information on line', to guide behavior by 'representational knowledge' is the essential function she attributes to the frontal cortex. Such a view appears to be consistent with the executive control function attributed to the frontal cortex in humans. In addition, this hypothesis begins to break down the concept of executive control into potentially separable subcomponents. Other recent research has emphasized the role of the frontal cortex in the registration of temporal order and frequency of occurrence information, stimulus attributes that are often encoded on an automatic basis in humans[31]. Thus the frontal cortex may mediate both complex, strategic cognitive processing as well as the more incidental and automatic forms of encoding. Given the qualitative differences between automatic-incidental encoding as compared with strategy selection and hypothesis testing, it seems altogether likely that different anatomical regions within the frontal cortex or different aspects of frontal–posterior cortex connectivity subserve these functions.

There have been multiple demonstrations of impaired WCS performance in patients with schizophrenia[32-34]. A dramatic example of the extent of the impairment was seen by Goldberg et al.[35] who attempted to incrementally teach patients to perform the test. They found that subjects were unable to benefit from explicit explanations of test conditions but were able to follow card by card instruction. However, when this instruction was eliminated, the patients returned to their impaired baseline performance level. Thus patients could not perform the test initially, an expected finding; they also could not learn how to perform the test, suggesting a true inability and profound compromise of prefrontal cognitive function. The cognitive operation that is responsible for the deficit remains unspecified as the WCS does not easily lend itself to an analysis of specific cognitive components because the stimulus displays are complex and response possibilities are multiple.

In an effort to simplify task demands, we recently developed a task which combines aspects of delayed response and delayed alternation. The task requires that the subject simultaneously track stimulus location and the regularly alternating correct response sequence. Only two stimulus locations and two response buttons are involved so that if a subject makes an error there is only one other possible response. It appears that the task imposes a significant load on working memory as adequate performance demands the continuous updating of the stimulus configuration and response sequence. In a pilot study, we have found that patients with schizophrenia have great difficulty with this task, with a majority performing at chance levels (Gold, unpublished data). More importantly, most patients continued to perform at chance after the rules of the task have been explained and they have been coached through a series of trials. This suggests that the striking abnormalities documented by Goldberg on the WCS may also be present on a very different task which is also thought to tax prefrontal function and require 'working memory'.

Deficits among schizophrenic patients have also been observed on a wide variety of tasks linked to frontal function such as verbal fluency, Trails B which requires repeated set alternation, on measures of abstracting ability such as the Category Test[36] and on simple graphomotor sequencing tasks where some patients demonstrate striking perseverative tendencies[37]. We have also recently found that patients with schizophrenia perform poorly on frequency estimation tasks and demonstrate an increased susceptibility to interference in a version of Wickens[38] release from proactive interference paradigm (Gold, unpublished data). The patients also had difficulty in temporal order discrimination as they intruded items from prior trials in the Wickens paradigm as well as in a separate verbal learning experiment which utilized three different lists presented consecutively. Thus, impairments have been observed both in effortful and strategic operations as well as in the more automatic processing of contextual information, suggesting a fundamental abnormality in frontal lobe function.

The more difficult interpretive issue is whether the impairments observed on frontally mediated tasks among patients with schizophrenia are differential deficits or are simply one aspect of a generalized deficit syndrome. There is certainly a great deal of evidence that schizophrenic patients perform abnormally on a wide array of cognitive tests, including tests which are not primarily mediated by the frontal cortex. In fact, it is often difficult to distinguish the neuropsychological test performance of chronic schizophrenic subjects from that of diffusely brain-damaged subjects[28a,38a].

This generality of deficits was recently highlighted in a study of MZ twins discordant for schizophrenia. In this study, Goldberg et al.[39] found that the affected twin performed more poorly than their unaffected co-twin on a wide range of neuropsychologial measures including tests of attention, memory, fluency, hypothesis testing, and motor speed. Remarkably, the ill twins performed at similar levels as their well counterparts on measures of motor learning and on Tower of Hanoi-type tasks, which appear to demand both conscious problem-solving as well as the operation of procedural memory which has been linked to the basal ganglia. The twin data demonstrate that cognitive impairment is present in nearly every case when a well twin is available as a control, although the extent of impairment may vary widely from one twinship to another. That is, even when an affected twin performed within the normal range on a given test, their well twin most often performed at higher levels. Thus, cognitive impairment is not limited to a subgroup of patients. Similarly, impairment is not seen only on one or two cognitive measures which are specific markers of the illness; the between twin differences are more striking and consistent on some measures than others, but on nearly every measure the unaffected twin outperformed the affected twin. This fact must temper any attempt at a strict localization of cognitive dysfunction in schizophrenia. Some cognitive operations appear to be more dysfunctional than others, implicating certain neural systems. However, even in the relatively spared cognitive operations it is hard to argue that performance is truly normal; the unaffected twins nearly always perform at higher levels.

It is unlikely that frontal dysfunction alone can easily account for the range of deficits seen in the twin study. There were clear, large differences in memory performance which may implicate temporal lobe dysfunction. Indeed, memory deficits are among the most frequently replicated findings in cognitive studies of schizophrenic patients[40]. In fact, the cognitive abnormalities may extend even beyond these structures as it is difficult to localize the frequently observed deficits in attentional processes[41]. Recent conceptualizations of the neural structures subserving attention have emphasized that wide spread areas of the cortex as well as subcortical centers may be involved, with different functions being subserved in different areas or combinations of areas[42]. Thus the neuropsychological data, as with the previous discussion of symptomatic variables, suggest that, while schizophrenia involves both frontal and temporal lobe dysfunction, these regions do not appear to account for the whole pattern of performance. One additional caveat should be mentioned in the interpretation of neuropsychological data. Neuropsychological localization is based on the study of the effect of focal lesions in adult patients.

The possibility cannot be excluded that developmental injuries such as may occur in schizophrenia might result in novel patterns of performance.

Frontal physiological hypofunction in schizophrenia

Studies of brain metabolism using positron emission tomography (PET) and regional cerebral blood flow (rCBF) techniques offer one method of validating the results of neuropsychological paradigms. We would suggest that the combination of abnormal task performance coupled with abnormal brain metabolism while performing a particular task sheds basic light on which brain regions and cognitive operations are qualitatively altered in the illness. This does not imply that poor performance coupled with normal metabolic activation signifies a cognitive deficit that is epiphenomenal or that the brain regions in question function normally. In this latter case, the evidence is more of a quantitative difference in the performance capability of a particular brain region rather than a true qualitative shift in the nature of the regional brain activity that is marshaled to meet a particular cognitive demand. We would expect that the routes to cognitive failure may be different in these two types of situations.

The most consistent evidence of abnormal metabolism coupled with abnormal performance has come from the NIMH studies of rCBF during the Wisconsin Card Sort[42a,45,46,49]. In these studies on four separate populations, metabolic activation has been studied by comparing the pattern of brain metabolic activity during the WCS to an active sensorimotor control task which requires perceptual matching. The control task makes similar perceptual and motor demands as the WCS but does not impose the need to abstract and test hypotheses. By subtracting the control task brain activity map from the WCS map, the task specific regional activation is highlighted. In normal controls, the WCS elicits activation of the dorsal lateral prefrontal cortex, consistent with the lesion data originally published by Brenda Milner[29]. In the NIMH studies, four different patient samples have demonstrated a failure to activate the DLPFC during the WCS, and this has been observed in both medicated and unmedicated groups. In all four studies patient performance on the task was deficient. It is important to note that the patients did not demonstrate hypofrontality during the control matching task; the between group difference emerged under the specific cognitive task condition that demands frontal activation. This was most striking in the study of discordant monozygotic twins: in every twin pair, the affected twin had reduced prefrontal rCBF during the WCS compared with their healthy co-twin[44]. This consistent finding of frontal hypometabolism during the WCS stands in contrast to the mixed results that have appeared in the literature concerning frontal metabolism in schizophrenic patients in the resting state[45].

While 'hypofrontality' has been reported in the resting state in some studies, the findings have been contradictory, suggesting that the most reliable method of assessing brain metabolism is to establish control over the mental activity that is occurring at the time of the scan.

In contrast to the WCS, patients with schizophrenia demonstrated normal patterns of frontal cerebral rCBF during the Ravens Progressive Matrices, a difficult nonverbal reasoning task[43]. The patients performed poorly on the task, but they activated the same posterior cortical areas as did normal controls. This finding suggests that it is not simply task difficulty or poor task performance per se that is responsible for the finding of hypofrontality on the WCS. Instead, it is most plausible to attribute these metabolic differences to the types of cognitive processing that the two tasks demand. The WCS demands active abstraction, hypothesis testing, and the use of feedback. The correct principle or feedback about prior incorrect responses must be retained and then serve to guide the selection of the next response. The Ravens also demands the abstraction of relationships between numerous stimuli. However, these stimuli are available for inspection and reinspection as the subject chooses a response. Each item is independent and the solution to one problem has no bearing on the next. It is the working memory dimension that may best distinguish the two tasks, and it is the working memory dimension that may be the critical determinant of prefrontal activation.

In the NIMH series of studies, schizophrenic patients also demonstrated normal prefrontal activity during the Continuous Performance Test (CPT)[42]. However the patients did demonstrate a different pattern of hemispheric activation: normal controls primarily activated the right hemisphere during the CPT X detection condition, whereas patients activated on the left[46]. Two other groups have also studied vigilance paradigms with concurrent metabolic imaging in patients with schizophrenia. Cohen et al.[47] reported frontal hypometabolism during a simple auditory attention task, and Buchsbaum et al.[48] reported frontal as well as right-sided temporal-parietal abnormalities during a degraded stimulus visual CPT. These studies are not easily comparable, as different tasks and imaging techniques were involved. The study of metabolic activity related to attentional processes is particularly complicated because it is unclear what the appropriate active control condition should be for vigilance tasks. That is, an active control task such as the number matching condition used in the WCS studies may control for too much of the variable of interest when studying attention. Alternately, simple visual stimulation with button pressing may approach the resting state in that considerable intrasubject variability in mental activity must be assumed. Despite these caveats, there is some tentative support for a coupling of abnormal performance and metabolism during sustained attention tasks in patients with schizophrenia. In light of the prominent role of attentional dysfunction in schizophrenia, these results suggest a basic qualitative deficit in the organizaton of brain metabolic activity during attentional processing. It is likely that these abnormalities extend beyond the frontal lobe. Further study and replication of these results are clearly needed before the attentional data can be understood.

At present, the metabolic imaging data suggest that hypofrontality is not the sole abnormality to be found in patients with schizophrenia. Further, the fact that frontal hypometabolism has not been consistently replicated in studies of the resting state raises the possibility that the failure to activate on cognitive demand results from a failure outside of the frontal lobe itself. Damaged brain tissue is generally hypometabolic whether studied at rest or under a cognitive load. This does not appear to be the case, or at least is not consistently the case, in patients with schizophrenia. The DLPFC activation failure in the context of frequently normal resting baseline suggests that the problem may lie in some aspect of the connectivity of the frontal cortex rather than intrinsic to the cortex itself[49].

To summarize, we have argued that many of the symptomatic, neuro-psychological, and metabolic findings in schizophrenia suggest a basic compromise of frontal function. However, in each of these areas it is clear that extra-frontal forms of dysfunction are probably implicated as well. We would suggest that frontal dysfunction is a necessary aspect of the illness, but is probably not sufficient to explain the wide array of behavioral, cognitive, and metabolic abnormalities that have been observed in patients with schizophrenia. In our view, the structural brain imaging and post-mortem findings to be discussed next are consistent with the hypothesis that frontal lobe dysfunction results from abnormalities in a series of different brain areas, many of which project to the frontal cortex. Thus the frontal cortex may be the brain area that most fully reflects the wide variety of subtle impairments that have been reported to date.

Anatomical neuropathology in schizophrenia

There have been literally hundreds of studies of post-mortem neuro-pathology, neurochemistry, and of anatomical brain imaging in patients with schizophrenia which cannot be adequately reviewed in the context of this chapter[2,3,50,51]. The neuropathological literature on schizophrenia from the early to mid part of this century defies easy summary. The literature is characterized by numerous findings of abnormalities throughout the brain including the frontal and temporal cortex, basal ganglia, brainstem, and limbic structures[50]. Many of these findings remain unreplicated or were sub-sequently contradicted by other studies. This inconsistency might be expec-ted in light of the lack of operational diagnostic criteria and the use of different examination techniques. The erratic nature of the research literature led some researchers to conclude that only coincidental factors had been uncovered. While this is undoubtedly partially true, the fact that recent neuroimaging results have consistently revealed structural brain abnormalities suggests that these early reports contained a true signal that was nearly hidden by the noise of methodological confounds. That signal is that brain abnormalities occur in a significant number of, if not all, patients with schizophrenia.

The original publication by Johnstone and colleagues in 1976 documenting enlargement of the lateral ventricles in schizophrenia visualized with the then newly available computed tomographic scanning technique opened a new chapter in the study of schizophrenia. In the following 15 years over a hundred similar studies have been published and several findings have reliably emerged[51]. First, enlargement of the ventricular system is now established as one of the critical pieces of evidence that schizophrenia involves direct alteration of brain structure. Lateral ventricular enlargement has been observed from centers around the world studying widely varying patient samples, although it should be noted that some negative results have been reported. This increase in brain CSF space is thought to reflect a reduction of brain tissue. While the ventricles are bounded by the basal ganglia, thalamus, limbic structures, and subcortical white matter, ventricular enlargement may be reflective of tissue loss at some distance from the ventricles and directly adjacent neural structures. Thus, this finding is not suggestive of any distinct type of focal brain abnormality.

The evidence accumulated to date suggests that these neuroanatomic changes cannot be attributed to the effects of somatic treatment and do not appear to be progressive, although this question warrants further study with MRI techniques[3,51].

There have also been multiple reports of enlargement of the third ventricle which is bounded by the hypothalamus, thalamus, and limbic forebrain nuclei as well as a number of major fiber tracts[51]. Thus, changes in the ventricular system are certainly suggestive of alterations in limbic, diencephalic, and basal ganglia structures if one makes the simplifying assumption that neighboring structures are likely to at least partially contribute to the effect.

There is also evidence that widespread areas of the cortex may be altered in the illness. This issue has been approached in the CT literature through measures of cortical fissures and markings, which if dilated are thought to reflect shrinkage of the underlying gyri. Reduced volume of the frontal and temporal cortex have been implicated with this method[53,54]. While the CT literature may offer some support for focal frontal structural abnormality, this has not been found in several MRI volumetric studies[1,55] although positive reports have appeared[56,57]. Several recent post-mortem investigations have also suggested frontal lobe pathology, including a loss of neurons and gyral irregularities[58,59]. Moreover, several groups have reported alterations in glutamate and $5\text{-}HT_2$ binding in the prefrontal cortex of post-mortem tissue from patients with schizophrenia[60,61]. The changes described to date appear to be relatively subtle and it is not surprising that these may not be reflected in volumetric imaging studies. Thus, while the possibility that structural abnormalities exist in the frontal cortex has not been established in a convincing fashion, such abnormalities cannot be ruled out on the basis of the current evidence and appear to exist according to some studies. It is clear, however, that pathology is by no means limited to the frontal cortex.

Recently, there have been several independent reports of changes in temporal lobe structures as visualized with MRI. This includes the report of Suddath et al.[1] which found evidence of a bilateral reduction of temporal lobe grey matter, Johnstone et al.[62] reported enlargement of the temporal horn of the lateral ventricles, and Bogarts et al.[13] who reported changes in the posterior component of the amygdala/ hippocampal complex in first break patients. The study of Suddath et al.[1] is especially intriguing because the reduction in hippocampal size predicted the enlargement in the ventricles. Perhaps the most compelling evidence for hippocampal pathology has come from the NIMH study of discordant MZ twins. In 14 of 15 cases the affected twin had decreased left anterior hippocampal area, while in 13 of 15 it was decreased on the right side[64]. Thus, when compared to an ideal control case, nearly every patient demonstrates hippocampal abnormalities, as was also found in the examination of ventricular size. The inconsistencies about which aspect of the hippocampus is most affected awaits further research.

One major reason that the finding of temporal lobe abnormalities on MRI has generated considerable interest is that recent post-mortem findings also implicate the same brain region. Bogerts et al.[65] reported volumetric reductions in the amygdala, hippocampal formation, and parahippocampal gyrus. Abnormalities have also been reported in reduced cell counts in the entorhinal cortex[66], in the width of the parahippocampal gyrus[67], and architectural abnormalities in the entorhinal cortex[68]. These findings have emerged from several different centers around the world using different brain collections.

This consistency between MRI-derived measurements of living patients and post-mortem studies is an important landmark in the study of schizophrenia. It should be noted that abnormalities in the other brain regions have also been described in recent post mortem studies such as the medial pallidum[65], and diffuse volumetric reduction of both grey and white matter[69]. It remains for future studies to determine to what extent these other abnormalities can be incorporated into a model of primary temporal lobe abnormality with secondary changes in afferent and efferent projection systems. Alternately, it cannot be ruled out that the temporal volumetric changes are secondary, and that given the crudity of current anatomical methods, primary changes in complex neocortex are less easily appreciated than are changes in archicortical and less-complex structures such as the hippocampus and entorhinal cortex.

J M Gold & D R Weinberger

At the present time structural abnormalities appear to be most reliably present in the medial temporal lobe. However, changes in subcortical structures as well as focal frontal abnormalities continue to be reported in the current literature. This again suggests that schizophrenia may involve multiple brain sites. Such a conclusion is also consistent with post-mortem neurochemical findings as reviewed by Hyde et al.[2]. They note reports of temporal lobe abnormalities include increased dopamine concentrations in the left amygdala, reduced cholecystokinin, somatostatin, and glutamate binding. There are also contradictory reports of alterations in D2 receptors in the basal ganglia, serotonin abnormalities in the globus pallidus, increased norepinephrine in the nucleus accumbens, and increased glutamate receptors in the frontal cortex, among many other positive findings. It should be noted that many of the neurochemical findings to date remain either unreplicated or disputed, and the interpretation of all such data is complicated by patient drug history. The important point is that the neurochemical abnormalities appear to be widespread, suggesting that a set of neural systems may be compromised in schizophrenia. As with the neuropathological literature, there is some evidence of direct alterations of frontal neurochemistry, but findings are by no means limited to the frontal cortex.

Schizophrenia: a disorder of Prefrontal–temporolimbic connectivity?
Clinical, neuropsychological, rCBF and PET, post-mortem, CT, and MRI studies are all consistent with the notion that the pathology of schizophrenia involves areas outside of the frontal cortex. However, the functional impact of these abnormalities may be maximal at the level of the frontal cortex. Indeed there is some direct evidence that this is the case. Berman et al.[70] found that ventricular enlargement correlated negatively with prefrontal activation only during the WCS. Similarly, Weinberger et al.[71] found that HVA and HIAA concentrations in CSF correlated with frontal activation, again only during the WCS. More recently, we have found in the study of MZ twins that the difference in anterior hippocampal size within a discordant twin pair strongly predicts the difference in prefrontal rCBF during the WCS (Weinberger, unpublished data). Thus the effect of presumably subcortical structural pathology and reductions in dopamine and serotonin metabolism is maximized when a specific cognitive demand is placed on the DLPFC.

Elkhonon Goldberg[72] has argued that the frontal lobe is likely to be compromised by extra-frontal lesions, given the extensive connectivity of the frontal cortex. Neuropsychologically, it is thought that the most complex forms of cognitive activity which are typically acquired late in development are the most vulnerable to nearly any type of brain injury. In essence, skills last to develop are the first to go. He has suggested that even truly diffuse brain injuries may often mimic focal frontal lesions. This is certainly a plausible hypothesis in light of the findings that we have reviewed in this chapter.

However this hypothesis may have difficulty accounting for several important aspects of the type of brain dysfunction that is seen in schizophrenia and the manner in which this abnormality comes to be apparent.

Many researchers have highlighted premorbid behavioral abnormalities in children at genetic risk for schizophrenia or in the developmental histories of adult schizophrenic patients[73]. While these early signs of compromise exist in some cases, many patients function fairly normally in most domains throughout early childhood. The behavioral difficulties evident in the early premorbid histories of even the poor premorbid cases rarely approaches the level seen in children with frank brain injuries. That is, the poor premorbid patients more closely approximate their age peers as children than they do when they are examined after the illness has developed. Thus, there is little evidence of moderately severe diffuse brain dysfunction during the developmental period in most cases. The onset of the illness appears to be coincident with a true worsening of brain functional capability. This occurs without evidence of an acute neurologic event, implying that the deterioration occurs more as a result of a potentiation of a previously subtle, if not largely silent vulnerability rather than as a de nouveau event. Goldberg's[72] caution that diffuse brain injuries may mimic those seen following frank frontal injuries is well taken, and the application of models of brain function based on the study of adult patients with focal lesions to the study of disorders with a presumed developmental origin is potentially problematic. However, this caution may be too broadly stated to pertain to schizophrenia; if the frontal syndrome of schizophrenia is truly only the result of diffuse cerebral dysfunction, then some developmental factor must be identified that could be responsible for the development of such a state.

Weinberger[74] has speculated that this type of potentiation model may fit the fact that the frontal cortex is a late-maturing brain region, and there is primate data supportive of the idea that an early developmental frontal lesion may only have its full behavioral impact following the normal development of cerebral functional specialization[75].

This line of reasoning can be most simply realized with intrinsic frontal damage. Can it be reconciled with the possibility that the temporal lobe may be the primary site of dysfunction, and that it is the temporal lobe that may present direct evidence of developmental compromise as has been suggested by several studies? The medial temporal and frontal lobes share direct bi-directional projections as well as indirect routes through the thalamus. There is evidence from the nonhuman primate that the performance of working memory tasks results in the metabolic activation of hippocampal, thalamic, as well as prefrontal structures[76-78]. Thus there is every reason to believe that a compromise of the medial temporal lobe may have an impact on the frontal cortex, and this may become most apparent with maturation. One direct example of such an effect has been reported by Hermann et al.[79] who observed that a substantial number of patients with temporal lobe epilepsy had difficulties performing the WCS, an abnormality that improved following temporal lobectomy. In that sample, abnormal activity in the temporal lobe appears to have produced a reversible compromise of prefrontal cognitive function.

It is somewhat unlikely that this is the full explanation for the frontal lobe syndrome in patients with schizophrenia. Some compromise of other frontal inputs would also be expected in light of the evidence of basal ganglia (i.e. medial pallidum) and ascending monoaminergic neurons involvement in the illness. One route to prefrontal compromise of extrinsic origin would be an abnormality in ascending dopamine projections which originate in the VTA. It seems implausible to suggest that this brainstem structure functions as the critical switch for the frontal cortex. That is, it is unlikely that a brainstem structure plays such a critical computational role in determining cortical activity. Instead, the role of ascending catecholamines seems to be to enhance the processing of the cortex, to help focus activity, and this input may be recruited by the cortex in a parallel fashion. On a more speculative note, it is possible that a failure of frontal metabolic activation could also result from a subtle intrinsic frontal abnormality which compromises the ability of the cortex to recrut inputs from connected brainstem and limbic structures.

Conclusion

The advances in the understanding of schizophrenia in the past 15 years can be largely attributed to the application of new techniques developed in the clinical and basic neurosciences. The findings to date clearly suggest that schizophrenia involves a basic compromise of brain structure and function. These abnormalities may be maximally expressed in the compromise of frontal lobe function, although the most consistently observed neuroanatomic defect in the illness appears to be in the temporal lobe. Further progress in the basic neuroscientific understanding of developmental processes, the role of dopamine, and anatomical connectivity will be necessary before it is possible to fully delineate the pathophysiology of the illness.

References

(1) Suddath RL, Casanova MF, Goldberg TE, Daniel DG, Kelsoe JR, Weinberger DR. Temporal lobe pathology in schizophrenia: a quantitative magnetic resonance imaging study. *Am J Psychiat* 1989; 146: 464–72.

(2) Hyde TM, Casanova MF, Kleinman JE, Weinberger DR. (in press). Anatomical and Neurochemical findings in schizophrenia. *Ann Rev Psychiat*.

(3) Zigun JR, Weinberger DR. (in press). In vivo studies of brain morphology in schizophrenia. In Linenmeyer J-P, Kay SR, eds. *New biological vistas on schizophrenia*. New York: Brunner Mazel.

(4) Levin S, Yurgelun-Todd D, Craft S. Contributions of clinical neuropsychology to the study of schizophrenia. *J Abnormal Psych* 1989; 98: 341–56.

(5) Seidman LJ. Schizophrenia and brain dysfunction: An integration of recent neurodiagnostic findings. *Psych Bull* 1984; 94: 195–235.
(6) Crow TJ. Molecular pathology of schizophrenia: more than one dimension of pathology? *Br Med J* 1980; 280: 66–8.
(7) Kraepelin E. *Dementia praecox and paraphrenia*. Melbourne, Florida: Robert E Krieger Publishing Co, Inc: 1971.
(8) Harlow JM. Recovery from the passage of an iron bar through the head. *Pub Mass Med Soc* 1868; 2: 327–46.
(9) Eslinger PJ, Damasio AR. Severe disturbance of higher cognition after bilateral frontal lobe ablation: Patient EVR. *Neurology* 1985; 35: 1731–41.
(10) Blumer D, Benson DF. Personality changes with frontal and temporal lobe lesions. In: Benson DF, Blumer D, eds. *Psychiatric aspects of neurologic disease*. New York: Grune & Stratton, 1975.
(11) Stuss DT, Benson DF. *The frontal lobes*. New York: Raven Press, 1985.
(12) Luria AR. *Higher cortical functions in man*. 2nd ed. New York: Basic Books, 1980.
(13) Norman DA, Shallice T. Attention to action. In: Davidson RJ, Schwartz GE, Shapiro D, eds. *Consciousness and self regulation* vol. 4. New York: Plennum Press, 1986.
(14) Sommers AA. Negative symptoms: conceptual and methodological problems. *Schizophrenia Bull* 1985; 11: 364–79.
(15) Carpenter WT Jr, Heinrichs DW, Alphs LD. Treatment of negative symptoms. *Schizophrenia Bull* 1985; 11: 440–52.
(16) Walker E, Levine RJ. The positive/negative symptom distinction in schizophrenia. *Schizophrenia Res* 1988; 1: 315–28.
(17) Levin S. Frontal lobe dysfunction in schizophrenia-II. Impairment of psychological and brain functions. *J Psychiat Res* 1984; 18: 57–72.
(18) Kapur N, Turner A, Kiha C. Reduplicative paraamneisa: possible anatomical and neurophysiological mechanisms. *J Neurol Neurosurg Psychiat* 1988; 5: 579–81.
(19) Stuss DT, Alexander MP, Lieberman A, Levine H. An extraordinary form of confabulation. *Neurology* 1978; 28: 1166–72.
(20) Pycock CJ, Kerwin RW, Carter CJ. Effect of lesion of cortical dopamine terminals on subcortical dopamine in rats. *Nature* 1980; 286: 74–7.
(21) Jaskiw GE, Weinberger DR. Ibotenic acid lesions of the medial prefrontal cortex potientiate FG-7142 induced attentuation of exploratory activity in the rat. *Pharmacol, Biochem, Behav* 1990; 36: 695–7.
(22) Stevens JR. An anatomy of schizophrenia? *Arch Gen Psychiat* 1973; 29: 177–89.
(23) Torrey EF, Peterson MR. Schizophrenia and the limbic system. *Lancet* 1974; ii: 942–6.
(24) Davison K, Bagley CR. Schizophrenia-like psychoses associated with organic disorders of the central nervous system. *Br J of Psychiat* 1969; 113 (suppl 1): 18–69.
(25) Penfield W, Rasmussen T. *The cerebral cortex of man*. New York: MacMillan Co, 1950.
(26) Gloor P, Olivier A, Quesney LF, Andermann F, Horowitz S. The role of the limbic system in experiential phenomena of temporal lobe epilepsy. *Ann Neurol* 1982; 12: 129–44.

(27) Halgren E, Walter RD, Cherlow DG, Crandall PH. Mental phenomena evoked by electrical stimulation of the human hippocampal formation and amygdala. *Brain* 1978; 101: 83–117.

(28) Heaton RK. *Wisconsin card sorting test manual.* Odessa, Florida: Psychological Assessment Resources, 1981.

(28a) Heaton RK, Baade LE, Johnson KL. Neuropsychological test results associated with psychiatric disorders in adults. *Psych Bull* 1978; 85: 141–62.

(29) Milner B. Effects of different brain lesions on card sorting. *Arch Neurol* 1963; 9: 90–100.

(30) Goldman-Rakic PS. Circuitry of primate prefrontal cortex and regulation of behaviour by representational knowledge. In: Plum F, Mountcastel V, eds. *Handbook of physiology: the nervous system V.* Washington DC: American Physiological Society, 1987.

(31) Schacter DL. Memory, amnesia, and frontal lobe dysfunction. *Psychobiology* 1987; 15: 21–36.

(32) Fey ET. The performance of young schizophrenics and young normals on the Wisconsin Card Sorting Test. *J of Cons Psych* 1951; 15: 311–19.

(33) Kolb B, Whishaw IW. Performance of schizophrenic patients on tests sensitive to left or right frontal temporal or parietal function in neurological patients. *J Nerv Ment Dis* 1983; 171: 435–43.

(34) Malmo HP. On frontal lobe functions: psychiatric patient controls. *Cortex* 1974; 10: 232–7.

(35) Goldberg TE, Weinberger DR, Berman KF, Pliskin NH, Podd MH. Further evidence for dementia of the prefrontal type in schizophrenia. *Arch Gen Psychiat* 1987; 44: 1008–14.

(36) Goldberg TE, Kelsoe JR, Weinberger DR, Pliskin NH, Kirwin PD, Berman KF. Performance of schizophrenic patients on putative neuropsychological tests of frontal lobe function. *Internat J Neurosci* 1988; 42: 51–8.

(37) Bilder RM, Goldberg E. Motor perservations in schizophrenia. *Arch Clin Neuropsych* 1987; 2: 195–214.

(38) Malec J. Neuropsychological assessment of schizophrenia versus brain damage: a review. *J Nerv Ment Dis* 1978; 166: 507–16.

(38a) Wickens DD. Encoding categories of words: an empirical approach to meaning. *Psych Rev* 1970; 77: 1–15.

(39) Goldberg TE, Ragland JD, Torrey EF, Bigelow LB, Gold JM, Weinberger DR. Neuropsychological assessment of monozygotic twins discordant for schizophrenia. *Arch Gen Psychiat* 1991: in press.

(40) Koh SD. Remembering of verbal materials by schizophrenic young adults. In: Schwartz S, ed. *Language and cognition in schizophrenia.* Hillsdale: Lawrence Erlbaum, 1978.

(41) Nuechterlien KH, Dawson ME. Information processing and attentional functioning in the developmental course of schizophrenic disorders. *Schizophrenia Bull* 1984; 10: 160–203.

(42) Posner MI, Peterson SE. The attentional system of the human brain. *Ann Rev Neurosci* 1990; 13: 25–42.

(42a) Berman KF, Zec RF, Weinberger DR. Physiological dysfunction of dorsolateral prefrontal cortex in schizophrenia: II Role of medication, attention, and mental effort. *Arch Gen Psychiat* 1986; 43: 126–43.

(43) Berman KF, Illowsky BP, Weinberger DR. Physiologic dysfunction in dorsolateral prefrontal cortex in schizophrenia: IV. Further evidence for regional and behavioural specificity. *Arch Gen Psychiat* 1988; 45: 616–22.

(44) Berman KF, Torrey EF, Daniel DG, Weinberger DR. Prefrontal cortical blood flow in monozygotic twins concordant and discordant for schizophrenia. *Schizophrenia res* 1989; 2: 129.

(45) Weinberger DR, Berman KF. Speculation on the meaning of cerebral metabolic hypofrontality in schizophrenia. *Schizophrenia Bull* 1988; 14: 157–68.

(46) Berman KF, Weinberger DR. Lateralisation of cortical function during cognitive tasks: Regional cerebral blood flow studies of normal individuals and patients with schizophrenia. *J Neurol Neurosurg Psychiat* 1990; 53: 150–60.

(47) Cohen RM, Semple WE, Gross M, et al. Dysfunction in a prefrontal substrate of sustained attention in schizophrenia. *Life Sci* 1987; 40: 2031–9.

(48) Buchsbaum MS, Nuechterlein KH, Haier RJ, et al. Glucose metabolic rate in normals and schizophrenics during the continuous performance test assessed by positron emission tomography. *Br J Psychiat* 1990; 156: 216–27.

(49) Weinberger DR, Berman KF, Zec RF. Physiologic dysfunction of dorsolateral prefrontal cortex in schizophrenia: 1. Regional cerebral blood flow (rCBF) evidence. *Arch Gen Psychiat* 1986; 43: 114–25.

(50) Kirch DG, Weinberger DR. Anatomical neuropathology in schizophrenia: post-mortem findings. In: Nasrallah HA, Weinberger DR, eds. *The handbook of schizophrenia: vol 1: the neurology of schizophrenia*. Amsterdam: Elsevier Science Publishers, 1986.

(51) Shelton RC, Weinberger DR. Computerised tomography in schizophrenia: A review and synthesis. In: Nasrallah HA, Weinberger DR, eds. *Handbook of schizophrenia vol 1: the neurology of schizophrenia*. Amsterdam: Elsevier, 1986.

(52) Johnstone EC, Crow TJ, Frith CD, Husband J, Kreel L. Cerebral ventricular size and cognitive impairment in chronic schizophrenia. *Lancet* 1976; ii: 924–6.

(53) Shelton RC, Karson CN, Doran AR, Pickar D, Bigelow L, Weinberger DR. Cerebral structural pathology in schizophrenia: evidence for a selective prefrontal cortical defect. *Am J Psychiat* 1988; 145: 154–63.

(54) Weinberger DR, Torrey EF, Neophytides AN, Wyatt RJ. Structural abnormalities in the cerebral cortex of chronic schizophrenic patients. *Arch Gen Psychiat* 1979; 36: 935–9.

(55) Kelsoe JR, Cadet JL, Pickar D, Weinberger DR. Quantitative neuroanatomy in schizophrenia. *Arch Gen Psychiat* 1988; 45: 533–41.

(56) Andreasen N, Nasrallah H, Dunn V, et al. Structural abnormalities in the frontal system in schizophrenia. A magnetic resonance imaging study. *Arch Gen Psychiat* 1986; 43: 136–44.

(57) DeMyer MK, Gilmore RL, Hendrie HC, DeMyer WE, Augustyn GT, Jackson RK. Magnetic resonance brain images in schizophrenic and normal subjects: influence of diagnosis and education. *Schizophrenia Bull* 1988; 14: 21–37.

(58) Benes FM, Davidson J, Bird ED. Quantitative cytoarchitectural studies of the cerebral cortex of schizophrenics. *Arch Gen Psychiat* 1986; 43: 31–5.

(59) Jacob H, Backmann H. Gross and Histological criteria for developmental disorders in brains of schizophrenics. *J Roy Soc Med* 1989; 82: 466–9.

(60) Deakin JFW, Slater P, Simpson MDC, et al. Frontal cortical and left temporal glutamatergic dysfunction in schizophrenia. *J Neurochem* 1989; 52: 1781–6.

J M Gold & D R Weinberger

(61) Mita T, Hananda S, Nishino N, et al. Decreased serotonin S2 and increased dopamine D2 receptors in chronic schizophrenics. *Biol Psychiat* 1986; 21: 1407–14.

(62) Johnstone EC, Owens DGC, Crow TJ, et al. Temporal lobe structure as determined by nuclear resonance in schizophrenia and bipolar affective disorder. *J Neurobiol Neurosurg Psychiat* 1989; 52: 533–41.

(63) Bogerts B, Ashtari M, Degreef G, Alvir JMJ, Bilder RM, Lieberman JA. Reduced temporal limbic structure volumes on magnetic resonance images in first episode of schizophrenia. *Psychiat Res* 1990; 35: 1–13.

(64) Suddath RL, Chirstison GW, Torrey EF, Weinberger DR. Cerebral anatomical abnormalities in monozygotic twins discordant for schizophrenia. *N Engl J Med* 1990; 322: 789–94.

(65) Bogerts B, Meertz E, Schonfeldt-Bausch R (1985). Basal ganglia and limbic system pathology in schizophrenia: a morphometric study of brain volume and shrinkage. *Arch Gen Psychiat* 1985; 32: 784–91.

(66) Falkai P, Bogerts B, Rozumek M. Limbic pathology in schizophrenia: the entorhinal region – a morphometric study. *Biol Psychiat* 1988; 24: 515–21.

(67) Brown R, Colter N, Corselis JAN, et al. Postmortem evidence of structural brain changes in schizophrenia: differences in brain weight, temporal horn area, and parahippocampal gyrus compared with affective disorder. *Arch Gen Psychiat* 1986; 43: 36–42.

(68) Jacob H, Beckmann H. Prenatal developmental disturbances in the limbic allocortex in schizophrenics. *J Neural Transmiss* 1986; 65: 303–26.

(69) Pakkenberg B. Post-mortem study of chronic schizophrenic brains. *Br J Psychiat* 1987; 44: 660–9.

(70) Berman KF, Weinberger DR, Shelton RC, Zec RF. A relationship between anatomical and physiological brain pathology in schizophrenia: lateral cerebral ventricular size predicts cortical blood flow. *Am J Psychiat* 1987; 144: 1277–82.

(71) Weinberger DR, Berman KF, Illowsky BP. Physiologic dysfunction of dorsolateral prefrontal cortex in schizophrenia: III. A new cohort and evidence for a monoaminergic mechanism. *Arch Gen Psychiat* 1988; 45: 609–15.

(72) Goldberg E. Akinesia, tardive dysmentia, and frontal lobe disorder in schizophrenia. *Schizophrenia Bull* 1985; 11: 255–63.

(73) Watt NF, Anthony EJ, Wynne LC, Rolf JE. *Children at risk for schizophrenia: a longitudinal perspective*. New York: Cambridge University Press, 1984.

(74) Weinberger Dr. Implications of normal brain development for the pathogenesis of schizophrenia. *Arch Gen Psychiat* 1987; 44: 660–9.

(75) Goldman-Rakic PS, Isseroff A, Schwartz ML, Bugbee NM. The neurobiology of cognitive development. In: Mussen P, ed. *Handbook of child psychology: biology and infancy development*, 4th ed. vol 21, New York: Wiley, 1983.

(76) Bugbee NM, Goldman-Rakic PS. Functional 2-deoxyglucose mapping in association cortex: prefrontal activation in monkeys performing a cognitive test. *Soc Neurosci Abst* 1981; 7: 416.

(77) Friedman HR, Goldman-Rakic PS. Activation of the hippocampus and dentate gyrus by working memory: a 2-deoxyglucose study of the behaving rhesus monkey. *J Neurosci* 1988; 8: 4693–706.

(78) Friedman HR, Janas JD, Goldman-Rakic PS. Enhancement of metabolic

Frontal lobes and schizophrenia

activity in the diencephalon of monkeys performing working memory tasks: a 2-Deoxyglucose study in behaving rhesus monkeys. *J Cognitive Neurosci* 1990; 2: 18–31.

(79) Hermann BP, Wyler AR, Richey ET. Wisconsin Card Sorting Performance in patients with complex partial seizures of temporal lobe origin. *J Clin Exp Neuropsych* 1988; 10: 467–76.

59

Neurotransmitter system abnormalities associated with the neuropathology of Alzheimer's disease

D DEWAR

Introduction

There has been extensive study of neurotransmitter systems in the brains of patients with Alzheimer's disease, over the last 10–12 years. In spite of, or perhaps due to, the enormous investigative effort in this area, it is now obvious that there is no single neurotransmitter system abnormality which can be associated specifically with this condition. A wide spectrum of neuro-transmitter system changes is, perhaps, not surprising in view of the anatom-ical loci which are afflicted by the structural correlates of this disease, namely; plaques, tangles and neuronal loss. These lesions are found predominantly in cerebral cortex and hippocampus, although within the cortex as a whole there is some degree of regional variation with association cortices being more severely affected than primary sensory areas. Tangle formation and neuronal loss also occur in subcortical regions, such as basal forebrain and brainstem nuclei, which send afferent projections to cortex and hippocampus. It is precisely those brain regions which undergo morphological change in Alzheimer's disease in which neurotransmitter systems are most frequently and significantly altered and, while the temporal relationship between the appearance of morphological and neurochemical changes is not known, at present, the inextricable link between brain structure and function predicts that, to some degree, one will not occur without the other.

In studying the literature concerning neurotransmitter system changes in Alzheimer's disease, it has become apparent that there is often tremendous inconsistency between different studies of a particular neurochemical parameter. This is especially true for neurotransmitter receptors. Differences in methodological approaches may account for some of the observed dis-

All correspondence to: Dr D Dewar, Wellcome Surgical Institute and Hugh Fraser Neuroscience Laboratories, University of Glasgow, Garscube Estate, Bearsden Rd, GLASGOW G61 1QH, UK.

Cambridge Medical Reviews: Neurobiology and Psychiatry Volume 1
© Cambridge University Press

crepancies although this is not to say that any of these are incorrect. Rather, the degree of *local* morphological change is a crucial factor in determining the extent to which neurotransmitter systems are altered within a given brain region. For example, the number of neurones within a particular region must have a major impact on the number of receptors which are located on those cell membranes. Alternatively, disruption of normal cell function, as evidenced by the presence of intracellular tangles, may influence neurotransmitter synthesis and/or release and possibly also receptor numbers. There is enormous individual variation in the degree of morphological change within a given group of Alzheimer brains. For example, in a sample of 18 subjects, the number of large neurones in frontal cortex ranged from 50–400 per mm[21] while in a similar-sized sample numbers of plaques in this brain region ranged from 10–95 per mm^2 (observations in this laboratory). Such wide variation in neuropathological parameters means that patient selection may have a major impact on measurements of neurochemical variables, particularly so if data is obtained from small groups.

Two methodological points concerning the study of neurotransmitter systems in Alzheimer brains are raised by this link between these systems and the underlying brain structure. First is the way in which the results of such investigations are expressed. Transmitter levels and receptor numbers are commonly expressed as per weight of tissue or protein in the sample. However, if neurotransmitter or receptor loss is simply an accompaniment of tissue loss then it will appear as if there is no change, as the two measures decrease proportionally together. This leads to a second methodological consideration which is that more useful information is gained if different parameters are measured in the same tissue sample than if a single measurement is made in isolation. An ideal paradigm for such studies is to determine the extent of *local* neuropathology in the same tissue sample as neurotransmitter-related measurements are made.

The role of the cholinergic system
One of the earliest neurochemical defects to be reported in Alzheimer's disease was a loss, from cerebral cortex, of choline acetyltransferase (ChAT), the synthetic enzyme for acetylcholine[2-4] and this has been confirmed by numerous subsequent studies[5]. The major afferent cholinergic projections of the cerebral cortex and of the hippocampus arise in the basal forebrain; nucleus basalis of Meynert, diagonal band of Broca and medial septal nuclei[6]. Histological examination of these brain structures revealed a significant loss of neurones in Alzheimer's disease consistent with the observed cortical cholinergic hypofunction[7-10]. A significant finding which suggested a critical role for this cholinergic system in the pathophysiology of Alzheimer's disease was the correlation between cortical ChAT deficits and both the severity of dementia and the number of cortical plaques[11]. The concept of Alzheimer's

disease being attributable to dysfunction of ascending cholinergic systems was initially extremely attractive, particularly in view of the well-documented role of central cholinergic mechanisms in learning and memory processes[12,13]. However, the wealth of data generated in the decade subsequent to these earlier findings suggest that the disease process most probably originates in cortical, not subcortical regions, and that degeneration of the cholinergic system is only one of many neurotransmitter abnormalities which play a role in the production of dementia of the Alzheimer type.

All studies of basal forebrain neurones must take place at post-mortem when it could be assumed that the majority of patients have reached the end of stages of the disease. However, there is marked individual variation in the extent of cell loss in the basal forebrain nuclei[8,14]. In one group of patients, while all of them exhibited reduced ChAT in the cerebral cortex, only half of the group had concomitant losses of ChAT in the nucleus basalis[15]. Intracortical cholinergic systems make only a small contribution to total cortical enzyme measurements therefore cortical cholinergic deficits must originate in ascending projections from the basal forebrain. A shrinkage of neuronal perikarya, as opposed to a loss, in the basal forebrain as found by Pearson et al[16] would explain discrepancies between the extent of cortical and subcortical cholinergic deficits.

A correlation between the degree of neuronal loss in the subdivisions of the nucleus basalis and the number of plaques in the areas of cerebral cortex to which these regions project suggested a role for the degeneration of ascending systems in the pathogenesis of cortical plaques[8,17,18]. If this was the case then it is highly probable that plaques would be present in other brain areas to which the nucleus basalis projects. However, there are few if any plaques in thalamic nuclei which receive such projections while these lesions are more prevalent in other thalamic nuclei which do not receive afferents from basal forebrain nuclei[19]. Immunohistochemical studies have revealed that, as well as cholinergic elements[20,21], plaques also contain markers for other putative neurotransmitters such as GABA[22], neuropeptide Y[23] somatostatin[21,24,25] and substance P[24,26]. For the large part, these latter transmitters are contained in intracortical neurones suggesting that these systems, as well as cortical afferents, are involved in plaque pathogenesis. The idea that cortical cholinergic deficits result from a retrograde degeneration of neurones initiated at the axon terminal rather than from a primary degeneration of subcortical neurones is further supported by the finding that the degree of neuronal loss in the nucleus basalis was approximately equalled by that observed in other subcortical nuclei which also project to the cerebral cortex: dorsal raphe nuclei and locus coeruleus[14]. These latter projections contain serotonin and noradrenaline, respectively, and markers for both these transmitters are reduced in the cerebral cortex and hippocampus both post-mortem and in biopsy tissue[27-32]. In accordance with these neurochemical changes in cortex, the corresponding cells of origin for serotoninergic and noradrenergic afferent projections are reduced in number in their respective subcortical nuclei[14,33–37]. Within a group of histologically confirmed Alzheimer patients there were a number of cases which had levels of cortical ChAT activity which were similar to control values but which had a significant loss of neurones from locus coeruleus and a modest fallout from dorsal raphe nuclei[14].

A prerequisite of cholinergic dysfunction for the production of dementia is open to question in the light of evidence from other neurodegenerative and dementing conditions. Acetylcholine synthesis was similar to control values in fresh cortical biopsy samples taken from demented patients who lacked the morphological stigmata of Alzheimer's disease[38]. Both demented and mentally unimpaired subjects wth Parkinson's disease had reduced levels of cortical ChAT although the demented group did have deficits of greater severity than non-demented subjects[39,40]. The neurodegenerative condition, olivopontocerebellar atrophy, is not a dementing condition although patients with this disease have mild neuropsychological disturbances[41]. However, the magnitude of the cortical ChAT deficit observed in a group of these patients was of similar magnitude to that in Alzheimer's disease[42]. Conversely, the symptoms of dementia in 4 patients who had Pick's disease were not accompanied by substantial alterations in cortical ChAT[43] although in a separate study of 2 such patients a marked loss of neurones in the nucleus basalis was noted[44]. Pick's disease is characterized by severe pyramidal cell degeneration in frontal and temporal cortices while the morphological hallmarks of Alzheimer's disease, plaques and tangles, are rarely observed. The relationship between cognitive impairment in Alzheimer's disease and both cholinergic deficits and cortical morphology was examined in a comprehensive study of cortical biopsy tissue taken 1–8 years after the emergence of clinical symptoms. Severity of dementia correlated strongly with markers of pyramidal cell degeneration but only poorly with ChAT activity. Since cortical cell markers did not correlate with cholinergic activity, it was suggested that subcortical degeneration need not necessarily be a causal factor in cortical dysfunction. Rather it was concluded that the symptoms of Alzheimer's disease may be attributed largely to degeneration of the pyramidal cells in cerebral cortex[45].

Cortical neurotransmitter systems
The devastating effects on almost all aspects of cognitive function in Alzheimer's disease point to a disruption of cognitive processing at the highest level. The predilection of higher order polymodal cortical association areas, such as frontal and parietal lobes as well as the medial temporal lobe, for higher densities of plaques and tangles, compared to primary sensory and motor cortices, is in keeping with this[46–49]. Within the cytoarchitecture of affected cortical regions the initial impression of Tomlinson et al[50,51] that

plaques were concentrated in cortical layers III and V was subsequently confirmed by quantitative morphology[46,52]. Lewis et al[53] suggested a less specific laminar distribution of plaques but confirmed the findings of Pearson et al[47] that tangles are found predominantly in large pyramidal cells. A marked loss of cortical pyramidal neurones from layers III and V has been found in Alzheimer's disease particularly in frontal and temporal areas[1,54–57]. These large cortical cells furnish both long cortico-cortical association fibres and corticofugal projections to the thalamus, basal ganglia and brainstem. Such cortical disconnection must have a profound influence on cognitive function and, indeed, Neary et al[45] found that mental test performance correlated more highly with cortical neuronal loss than with plaque or tangle frequency and correlated only poorly with ChAT activity.

The major neurotransmitter utilized by pyramidal cells of both the cerebral cortex and the hippocampus is putatively the excitatory amino acid glutamate[58]. In addition to cortical associational input, these neurones also receive ascending projections from the basal forebrain (cholinergic), raphe nuclei (serotonergic) and brainstem (noradrenergic). Furthermore, a system of short cortical interneurones containing GABA and a number of different neuropeptides also impinge upon, and receive from, pyramidal cells[59]. Thus degeneration of pyramidal cells, as well as the formation of plaques and tangles, in Alzheimer's disease, must be associated with disturbances in a wide range of neurotransmitter systems within the cerebral cortex.

Glutamate receptors

There is substantial evidence demonstrating glutamatergic dysfunction in Alzheimer's disease, although biochemical measurements of glutamate levels in brain tissue are confounded by the participation of this amino acid in a variety of metabolic processes and thus only a proportion of free brain glutamate represents the neurotransmitter pool[60]. Probably as a consequence of this, studies of brain glutamate levels in Alzheimer brain have provided equivocal evidence as regards the status of glutamatergic neurones. Some studies report reduced glutamate levels in cerebral cortex and hippocampus at postmortem[61–65] while others report no change[66,67]. In biopsy material, the K^+-stimulated release of glutamate and aspartate was no different in Alzheimer patients compared to controls[68] although direct measurement of the levels of these putative neurotransmitters in biopsy samples have again proved inconclusive[65,67].

A more fruitful approach in assessing glutamatergic neurones in Alzheimer brain has been the use of markers which identify presynaptic glutamatergic terminals and postsynaptic glutamate receptors. [^{3}H]-D-aspartate, under the appropriate conditions, binds to a site on presynaptic glutamatergic terminals which is associated wth a high affinity glutamate uptake mechanism and this ligand serves as a useful marker for glutamatergic innervation[69]. In homogenates of cerebral cortex and hippocampus, [^{3}H]-D-aspartate binding was reduced by 30–60% of control values in Alzheimer brains[40,70-75]. Similarly, active uptake of [^{3}H]-D-aspartate into synaptosomal preparations was reduced by 50–70% in frontal, temporal, parietal and occipital cortices[76,77]. While such evidence suggests that there are certainly deficits of cortical and hippo-campal glutamatergic innervation in Alzheimer's disease there are certain discrepancies between some of these reports. For example, while Hardy et al[76] report reductions in active [^{3}H]-D-aspartate uptake of approximately 60% in frontal, parietal, temporal, occipital cortices and the hippocampus, Cow-burn et al[74] report that [^{3}H]-D-aspartate binding is reduced by 50% in temporal cortex, but it is similar to control values in frontal and parietal cortices. A similar discrepancy is apparent in two independent studies of parietal cortex in which [^{3}H]-D-aspartate binding was reduced by 60% in one study[72] but was unchanged in another[70]. This is not to suggest that any of these studies are incorrect and it is possible that methodological differences may account to some extent for discrepancies. However, what is not clear when making comparisons between these studies is the variation which may exist in the degree of *local* structure abnormalities (neuronal loss, plaques, tangles) within the individual brain regions examined. The wide variation in the densities of morphological abnormalities between individual patients and across brain regions[46,47,54] suggests that presuppositions about a constant regional pattern of glutamatergic presynaptic terminal loss in Alzheimer's disease are unfounded. Assuming that these terminals contribute to the for-mation of cortical plaques, is there any evidence for a correlation between glutamatergic terminal loss and plaque density within a given anatomical locus? Quantitation of these two parameters within the same tissue sample suggest not. Using quantitative autoradiography to measure [^{3}H]-D-aspartate binding in middle frontal cortex there was a 50% loss of glutamatergic ter-minals from all cortical layers in Alzheimer brains compared to controls (Fig. 1). However, there was no correlation between levels of [^{3}H]-D-aspartate binding and the number of plaques either in superficial (I–III) or deep (IV–VI) cortical layers[78]. This finding may not be surprising in view of the contribution which other neurotransmitters make to the formation of plaques (see previously). Charlton and colleagues[79] did not find a loss of [^{3}H]-D-aspartate binding from any cortical region in their quantitative autoradio-graphic study. However, it is not clear how the degree of local neuro-pathology in their samples compares with that in our study.

The two major sources of cortical glutamatergic innervation arise from pyramidal neurones in other areas of the cerebral cortex and from the thalamus[58]. Therefore, a deficit in cortical glutamatergic presynaptic ter-minals in Alzheimer's Disease may be associated with a concomitant loss of their cells of origin. Within the cortex, these cells, in turn, will themselves receive glutamatergic innervation and will express receptors for glutamate.

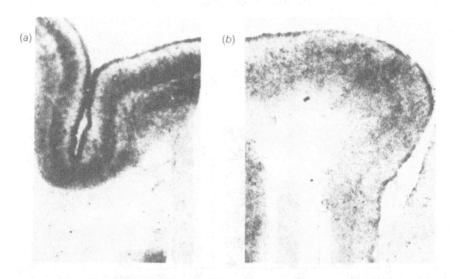

Fig. 1. Representative autoradiograms of [³H]-D-aspartate binding to presynaptic glutamatergic terminals in sections of frontal cortex in control (*a*) and Alzheimer (*b*) brain. Note the reduction in [³H]-D-aspartate binding throughout Alzheimer frontal cortex in comparison with control and the significant diminution in the prominence of the laminar pattern of binding in Alzheimer frontal cortex. From Chalmers et al[78].

These receptors can be subdivided into at least 3 distinct types on the basis of their sensitivity to the 3 agonists: *N*-methyl-D-aspartate (NMDA), kainate and quisqualate[80]. Kainate and quisqualate receptors are believed to be involved in classical, fast, synaptic transmission while the NMDA receptor and its associated voltage-dependent ion channel have been implicated in processes involved in learning and memory[81]. It is probably for ths reason that this latter subtype of glutamate receptor has been the focus of many investigations in Alzheimer's disease.

The initial autoradiographic study of glutamate receptors in Alzheimer's disease, by Greenamyre and colleagues[82], showed a 35–40% reduction in NMDA receptor binding in outer layers of temporal cortex compared to either non-demented controls or patients with Huntington's disease although this study has been criticized on methodological grounds[83,84]. This finding has not been replicated by studies using homogenate preparations of temporal cortex and either [³H]-MK-801 or [³H]-TCP, ligands which bind within the ion channel associated with the NMDA recognition site[73–75,85]. In contrast, however, there was a slight reduction (20%) in NMDA-sensitive [³H]-glutamate binding confined to the outermost cortical layers of frontal cortex (Fig. 2). Quantification of the number of plaques in tissue sections adjacent to those used for autoradiography revealed that both temporal and frontal cortex

D Dewar

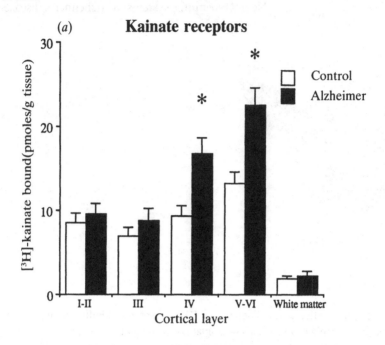

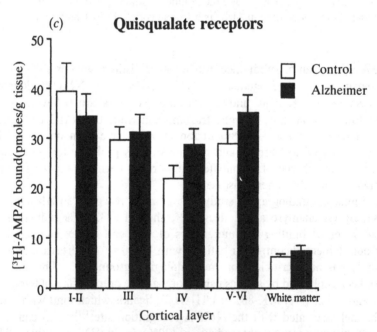

Fig. 2. Presynaptic glutamatergic terminals and postsynaptic glutamate receptors were labelled by means of quantitative ligand binding autoradiography in consecutive sections of frontal cortex from control and AD subjects. (a) [³H]-kainate binding; (b) [³H]-aspartate binding to presynaptic glutamatergic terminals; (c) [³H]-AMPA bind-

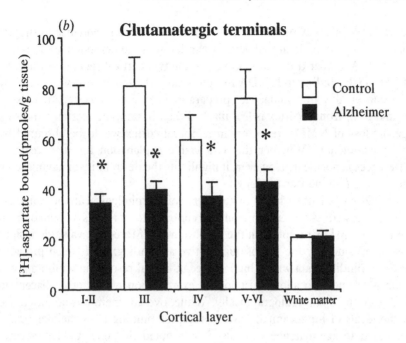

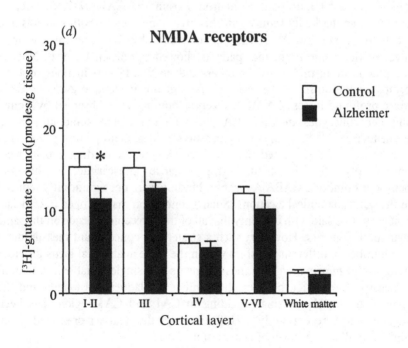

ing to quisqualate receptors; (*d*) NMDA-sensitive [³H]-glutamate binding. Data are mean ± SEM, *n*=6 for both groups. *p<0.05, student's t-test. From Chalmers et al[78].

had a similar density of these lesions. Moreover, there is evidence to suggest that the degree of neuronal loss is similar in both temporal and frontal cortices[1]. A similar difference between these two cortical regions in the level of [³H]-TCP binding to NMDA receptors in Alzheimer brains was found by Simpson et al[73], in homogenate preparations. It was suggested that tissue shrinkage in frontal cortex is less marked than in temporal cortex[55] and so a specific loss of NMDA receptors in temporal cortex would be obscured by this phenomenon. Whether this is a viable explanation for such regional differences is not clear. However, it highlights the desirability of having some measure of *local* neuropathology.

Individual patient variation in the degree of morphological abnormality has been suggested as an explanation for contradictory results obtained from studies of NMDA receptors in the hippocampus. Moreover, valuable insight has been gained by the use of quantitative autoradiography which provides receptor binding data with a high degree of spatial resolution within a given brain area and also allows histological examination of sections adjacent to those examined autoradiographically. While, overall, there was no difference in the levels of hippocampal NMDA receptor binding in Alzheimer brains compared to age-matched controls, it was noted that one Alzheimer case, which had a 50% dropout of neurones from the CA1, NMDA receptor binding was markedly reduced in this area compared to both controls and other Alzheimer cases[86]. A subsequent study, by the same investigators, revealed that some Alzheimer patients showed significant losses of NMDA receptor binding in CA1 while others did not[87]. Mean reductions of 40%, compared to control, were seen in CA1 but not in dentate gyrus or CA3. More profound losses of NMDA receptor binding were observed by Young and her colleagues in CA1, CA3, dentate gyrus and subiculum in all Alzheimer cases[88,89]. While direct measures of local neuropathology were not described, it was suggested that the NMDA receptor binding deficits were not simply due to tissue atrophy since muscarinic, cholinergic, benzodiazepine and GABA A receptor binding were not significantly reduced in the same anatomical locations. Such a conclusion may be open to criticism as it cannot be said with certainty that all of these receptors reside on the same structural elements. However, such a strategy of concomitant measurement of a number of different variables within the same anatomical locus provides more useful information than measurements of a single variable in isolation. A negative correlation between the number of plaques and tangles and the level of total [³H]-glutamate binding in CA1 and CA3 regions has been suggested in a recent study[90]. Unfortunately, the data set presented is too limited to allow any form of statistical analysis.

The anatomically discrete deficits in NMDA receptors, detected by the use of autoradiography, and their relationship to local neuropathology may explain why the use of homogenate preparations has demonstrated only modest reductions[73] or no change[65,74,75,77,85] in NMDA receptors in the hippocampus. A similar contrast between studies, using either whole tissue homogenates or autoradiography is seen in investigations of kainate receptors. No alteration in the level of kainate receptor binding was observed in homogenate preparations of frontal, temporal and parietal cortices or the hippocampus and caudate nucleus from Alzheimer brains[91]. However, using quantitative autoradiography, a significant increase (50%) in the level of kainate receptor binding was observed in deep layers IV–VI of frontal cortex while in superficial cortical layers I–III the level of binding was similar to controls (Figs 2 and 3). Such a laminar-specific increase in kainate receptor binding would probably have been obscured when a homogenate of the entire cortical grey matter was used. The increase in kainate receptor binding was closely associated with the degree of local structural change in that there was a positive correlation between the local number of plaques in cortical layers IV–VI and the level of kainate receptor binding in those layers (Fig. 4). There was no such correlation between kainate receptor binding and plaque densities in cortical layers I–III. Concurrent measurement of NMDA and quisqualate (AMPA) receptor binding and d-aspartate binding to presynaptic glutamatergic terminals, in adjacent sections to those used for kainate receptor binding, revealed a slight (20%) reduction in NMDA receptors (layers I–II), no change in quisqualate (AMPA) receptors and a significant (50%) loss of presynaptic glutamatergic terminals (layers I–VI) respectively (Fig. 1, 2 and 3). Although, at a simplistic level, it would be tempting to speculate that there was an upregulation of kainate receptors in response to presynaptic glutamatergic denervaion such a conclusion does not appear to be viable in view of the concomitant loss of presynaptic input, but preservation of kainate receptor binding, in layers I–III. The reason for a preservation of corticofugal information processing in the presence of intracortical glutamatergic dysfunction remains unclear at present.

Kainate receptor upregulation in the face of presynaptic denervation has been suggested in the hippocampus, in Alzheimer's disease where an expansion of the kainate receptor binding field was observed[92]. A similar phenomenon occurred in experimental animals following lesions of the entorhinal cortex, the major glutamatergic input to the hippocampus. Geddes et al[92] suggested that a similar situation exists in the Alzheimer brain, since, the large cells of the entorhinal area are lost. However, the density of kainate receptors was not quantified in their study, only the width of the binding field. A subsequent quantitative autoradiographic study of kainate receptor binding in the hippocampus, in a small number of Alzheimer cases, reported a marked decrease in the dentate gyrus, compared to age-matched controls. Although the small number of samples precluded statistical correlation analysis it appeared qualitatively, at least, that the cases which had the highest number of plaques and tangles had the lowest levels of kainate binding[90]. Finally, with regard to a possible upregulation of kainate receptors in response to a loss of glutamatergic input in the Alzheimer brain, it is interest-

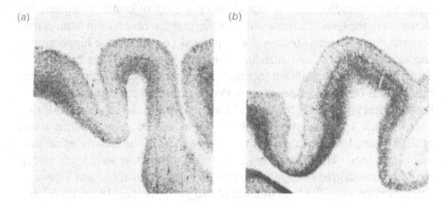

Fig. 3. Representative autoradiograms of kainate receptor binding in sections of frontal cortex in control (a) and Alzheimer (b) brain. In Alzheimer frontal cortex, kainate receptor binding is increased in deep cortical layers and unaltered in superficial cortical layers in comparison with control. From Chalmers et al[78].

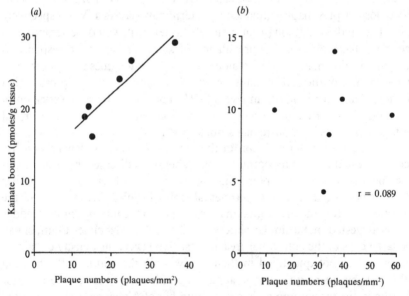

Fig. 4. Positive correlation between kainate receptor binding and plaque numbers in layers IV–VI of frontal cortex in AD. Kainate receptor binding was determined by means of quantitative autoradiography and plaques were quantified in tissue sections, from the same subjects no more than 0.5 cm caudal to those used for autoradiography. Data points represent individual AD subjects. From Chalmers et al[78].

ing to note that d-aspartate binding in the caudate nucleus, presumably reflecting descending glutamatergic input from the cerebral cortex, is reduced[73–75]. However, the lack of change in kainate receptor binding in the caudate[91,93] would argue against any denervation supersensitivity reaction, at least in this brain area.

Dysfunction of glutamatergic systems has been proposed as a possible mechanism involved in neuronal degeneration in Alzheimer's disease[94] and certain properties of glutamate have lent support to such a hypothesis. These include the involvement of NMDA receptors in learning and memory processes, particularly in the hippocampus[81,95], and the powerful neurotoxic actions of glutamate. With regard to the latter, glutamate neurotoxicity has been implicated in the neuronal death associated with conditions such as ischaemia, epilepsy and Huntington's disease[96]. Moreover, injection of NMDA into the cerebral cortex of rats gave rise to a retrograde degeneration of cholinergic neurones arising in the basal forebrain[97]. While the evidence is not suggestive of an etiological role for glutamate in Alzheimer's disease, it cannot be ruled out that glutamate dysfunction plays a role in the progression of the disease. As yet unknown factors, such as toxins or viral agents may initiate the pathophysiological process of the disease. However, glutamate neurotoxicity may hasten the progression of the degenerative changes.

Cholinergic receptors

Despite the extensive documentation describing the status of cortical muscarinic receptors in Alzheimer's disease no consistent changes are apparent. Reports of either reductions or no change in the number of cortical and/or hippocampal muscarinic receptors are approximately of equal numbers while there are a smaller number of studies describing increased numbers of receptors[5] Many of the less recent studies used the ligand [^{3}H]-quinuclidylbenzilate in binding assays which does not differentiate the two major muscarinic receptor subtypes, M_1 and M_2. There have been suggestions that discrepant results may be explained on the basis of a selectivity of muscarinic receptor subtype changes. Autoradiographic analysis of M_1 and M_2 muscarinic receptors in cerebral cortex[98] and hippocampus[99] revealed no significant alterations in either receptor. Subsequently, there were reports of a preservation of M_1 receptors with a concomitant substantial reduction in the number of M_2 sites[100,101]. However, others have reported only moderate reductions in M_2 receptors in the hippocampus[102,103] but not in frontal or temporal cortex[103]. There was also a small reduction in the number of M_1 receptors in the hippocampus, in one study[102], although others reported no change[103] or even a slight increase[101]. Thus, even when individual muscarinic receptors subtypes are examined, the evidence for change is equivocal.

Smith et al[102] highlight the variability in the number of hippocampal M_2 receptors in their Alzheimer patients, with numbers ranging from 0–50% of control values, and propose that M_2 receptors may be lost at later stages in the disease process. This suggestion gains credence from an elegant study in which the relationship between hippocampal muscarinic receptors and local neuropathology was examined in detail[104]. Quantitative ligand binding auto-radiography revealed no significant difference in either the densities of total muscarinic receptors, or the proportions of M_1 and M_2 subtypes, in the CA1 field of the hippocampus. Quantification of CA1 pyramidal cells in tissue sections adjacent to those used for autoradiography revealed a significant reduction in these cells in Alzheimer patients although there was wide individual variation. In those cases in which pyramidal cell loss was most severe, muscarinic receptor density was decreased compared to controls. Within the group as a whole there was a significant correlation between the number of neurones and the density of muscarinic receptors (Fig. 5a). More interestingly, however, the ratio of muscarinic receptors to pyramidal cell was increased in the Alzheimer patients (Fig. 5b). Thus, the suggestion was made that compensatory increases in hippocampal muscarinic receptors are poss-ible in intact neurones although beyond a certain threshold of local neuronal degeneration this compensatory response is no longer possible.

Whether such compensatory receptor increases respond to either neuronal fallout or presynaptic cholinergic hypofunction is at present unclear. However, unchanged levels of muscarinic receptors in the face of reduced levels of ChAT may suggest a receptor response to a loss of presynaptic input[105,106] as would an elevation in the number of hippocampal receptors with a concomitant loss of ChAT[107]. In this regard it is also worth noting that in patients with Parkinson's disease, who were not demented, a significant loss of cortical ChAT activity was accompanied by an increase in muscarinic receptors[102,108,109]. This cholinergic receptor denervation supersensitivity is supported by a negative correlation between the number of muscarinic receptors and the level of ChAT activity in the cerebral cortex of Parkinson's disease patients[103]. However, there is little experimental evidence from cholinergic lesioning studies to suggest that such a phenomenon occurs, at least in rodents[100,110,111].

The actions of acetylcholine are not only mediated by muscarinic receptors but also by nicotinic receptors. The status of these receptors is somewhat less controversial than the muscarinic type. By far the majority of studies report significant reductions in both cortex and hippocampus[112-117]. One report of unchanged nicotinic receptors[105] has been criticized for its use of unwashed membrane preparations as brain tissue contains a putative endogenous nicotinic receptor inhibitor[117]. Parallel reductions in the level of ChAT activity along with nicotinic receptor loss have suggested a presynaptic loca-tion for these receptors which is supported by the ability of nicotine to stimulate the release of acetylcholine[118]. However, lesions of the basal fore-brain in rodents resulted either in unaltered or increased numbers of nicotinic

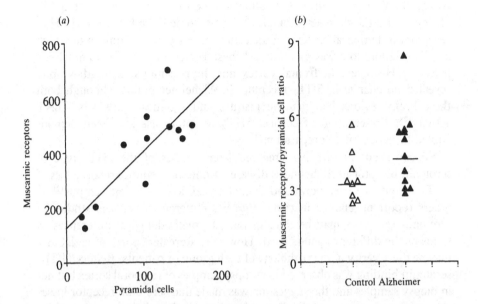

Fig. 5. (a) Relationship between numbers of hippocampal muscarinic receptors and pyramidal cells in Alzheimer brains. [³H]-N-methyl scopolamine binding to muscarinic receptors was determined in sections of hippocampus by means of quantitative autoradiography. Pyramidal cell numbers were determined in consecutive sections from the same brains. Data points represent individual AD cases. (b) Ratio of hippocampal muscarinic receptors to pyramidal cells. Data was derived as in (a) and is expressed as the number of muscarinic receptors per pyramidal cell in CA1. Mean ratios are indicated by the horizontal bars. Note the increased ratios of receptor/cell in AD subjects. Data redrawn from Probst et al[104] with kind permission.

receptors in cerebral cortex and hippocampus[119,120]. A pre- or postsynaptic location, on both, would explain the consistent loss of nicotinic receptors.

Serotonin receptors

A loss of serotonin receptors from cerebral cortex and hippocampus is one of the most consistent features of Alzheimer brain at post-mortem. Serotonin receptors can be divided into $5HT_1$, $5HT_2$ and $5HT_3$ subtypes and the $5HT_1$ subtype further divided into $5HT_{1A}$, 1B, and 1C. Of these subtypes, the $5HT_2$ receptor is most consistently and significantly reduced. Losses of $5HT_2$ receptors of up to 60% of control values have been reported in frontal[121–123], temporal[121,124] and parietal cortex[77,125] as well as in the hippocampus[121]. There is evidence to suggest that this loss of $5HT_2$ receptors reflects cortical pyramidal cell loss. The distribution of $5HT_2$ receptors within cerebral cortex, mapped by means of ligand binding autoradiography, indicates that these receptors are most prevalent in cortical layers III and V[126]. Neurofibrillary tangles are concentrated in the cells of layers III and V[47] and in entorhinal cortex there was an inverse relationship between the density of $5HT_2$ receptors and the number of tangles.[125] An autoradiographic study of $5HT_2$ receptors in temporal cortex revealed that there were two laminae in which $5HT_2$ receptors loss was greatest and these corresponded to pyramidal cell layers[127]. However, in frontal cortex and hippocampus, autoradiography revealed no change in $5HT_2$ receptors in Alzheimer brains, although both these brain regions had neuritic plaques and significant losses of ChAT activity[128]. Preservation of cortical $5HT_2$ receptors has also been demonstrated in homogenate preparations[129].

No consistent picture has emerged from studies of the $5HT_1$ type of serotonin receptor in Alzheimer's disease. While some studies report a loss of $5HT_1$ receptors in temporal and frontal cortex and the hippocampus[121,130] others report no change in cortex[123,124,127]. Differences between studies of serotonin receptors may be due, in part, to methodological differences in terms of the different ligands used. However, a greater source of variability may be the severity of the pathology of each group of patients. Reduced [^{3}H]-serotonin binding was observed in autopsy samples of temporal cortex but not in biopsy samples and the suggestion was made that serotonin receptor losses are not an early feature of the disease but rather follow the progression of the disease[29].

Adrenoreceptors

β-adrenoreceptors were preserved in temporal cortex, in Alzheimer brains, although in the same tissue samples, markers which reflect the integrity of neuronal membranes and perikarya, were reduced by approximately 25%[29]. Others have also reported unchanged levels of both β- and α-adrenoreceptors in both temporal and frontal cortex in Alzheimer's disease[121,124,131–133]. However, in the hippocampus, α_1 receptors were reduced while α_2 were unchanged and B_1 receptors were reduced while B_2 were increased[132,133]. Increased levels of B_2 receptors have recently been reported in prefrontal cortex, in Alzheimer's disease, while in the same tissue, B_1 receptors were decreased. Autoradiography revealed the increases in B_2 receptors to be localized to cortical layers II–V[134]. In the same patients, the level of noradrenaline in frontal cortex was reduced by approximately 50% and the number of cells in the locus coeruleus was also markedly reduced compared to controls. Increased numbers of B_2 and B_1 receptors were also observed in the hippocampus and Kalaria and colleagues[134] suggest that both cortex and hippocampus, in the Alzheimer brain, are capable of receptor plasticity, perhaps in response to a loss of presynaptic input.

Cortical interneuronal systems

Although there is morphometric data indicating a consistent loss of cortical pyramidal cells in Alzheimer's disease, there is little data of this sort concerning other types of cortical neurones, in particular short intrinsic interneurones. However, neurochemical and histochemical studies do suggest that certain populations of these neurones are lost.

γ-Aminobutyric acid (GABA) is believed to be the major inhibitory neurotransmitter of a number of intrinsic cortical interneurones and cortical GABA concentrations are reduced in Alzheimer's disease[135-137] although a number of other studies reported no change in the level of GABA-synthesizing, enzyme, glutamic acid decarboxylase[136-138]. However, it has been noted that the activity of this enzyme is influenced by premortem factors[139] and thus interpretation of such studies is complicated by the agonal state of individual patients[140,141]. The involvement of GABAergic neurones in cortical plaque formation is indicated by the presence of glutamic acid decarboxylase immunoreactivity in cortical plaques[22] and a loss of GABAergic innervation is suggested by reduced levels of GABA reuptake markers[142,143]. Consistent with these findings are reports of reduced concentrations of somatostatin[144-148] which is colocalized with GABA in non-pyramidal neurones[149]. The susceptibility of these neurones to the pathological process of Alzheimer's disease is further indicated by the presence of neurofibrillary tangles in somatostatin-containing neurones[150] and somatostatin-like immunoreactivity in plaques[148,151]. It has been suggested that changes in these short cortical neurones occur in the late stages of the disease process since cortical biopsy samples from Alzheimer patients released as much GABA[152] and somatostatin[153] as control samples and the levels of these two transmitters were not reduced in biopsy samples taken from patients 1-3 years after the onset of the disease[154]. The pattern of focal cortical hypometabolism, measured *in vivo* by positron emission tomography, in a group of patients 1-5 years after the onset of presumed Alzheimer's disease was paralleled by the distribution of somatostatin, but not ChAT, deficits in post-mortem tissue from a separate group of patients who were presumably at end stage[155]. However, there is no reason to exclude other focal structural or neurochemical abnormalities as factors contributing to the observed cortical hypometabolism since no other variables were measured. At a local level, somatostatin deficits appear to be linked closely to the severity of structural pathology as the loss of somatostatin neurones was greatest in regions of the temporal cortex which had the highest number of plaques and neurofibrillary tangles[148].

Cholecystokinin (CCK), vasoactive intestinal peptide (VIP), corticotrophin releasing factor (CRF) and neuropeptide Y (NPY) are also believed to be transmitters of cortical non-pyramidal neurones. There are conflicting theories as to the status of NPY concentrations in the cerebral cortex of Alzheimer patients[147,156,157]. However, immunocytochemical studies have demonstrated severe losses of NPY-containing neurones from temporal cortex and the hippocampus and while, in some cases these neurones are preserved, their morphology is abnormal[147,158]. NPY and somatostatin coexist in some cortical and hippocampal neurones and accordingly there was an equal loss of immunocytochemical markers for these two peptides in the hippocampus of patients described as 'severe', both clinically and pathologically[148]. VIP concentrations in cerebral cortex were either unchanged[159-161] or only modestly reduced[162]. Significant reductions in the concentration of CRF were found in cerebral cortex[163,164], although CRF immunoreactivity was preserved in the hippocampus[165]. Interestingly, the reduction in the level of CRF in occipital cortex was similar to that in frontal and temporal cortex[166]. Occipital cortex is generally regarded as being relatively spared, in terms of plaques and tangles, compared to other cortical regions. CCK and substance P levels were not consistently reduced in Alzheimer cerebral cortex, despite the colocalization of these peptides with GABA[161,167,168].

It is hardly surprising that receptors for these transmitters are altered in Alzheimer's disease, as a large proportion of these will be located on neuronal elements which are degenerating, e.g. presynaptic terminals, pyramidal cell perikarya and other intrinsic neurones. The actions of GABA are mediated by two distinct receptors subtypes, GABA A and GABA B. Audioradiographic analysis of these receptors in frontal cortex revealed marked reductions in the number of GABA B receptors localized in cortical layers III and V[169]. By contrast, GABA A receptors were only slightly reduced in these layers. These differential receptor deficits suggest that GABA A receptors are probably, for the most part, situated on cortical interneurones that are relatively spared in Alzheimer's disease. A population of GABA B receptors are probably located on pyramidal cells but the ability of GABA B receptor stimulation to alter the presynaptic release of glutamate, noradrenaline and serotonin also indicates a presynaptic location. A combination of pre- and post-synaptic degeneration could therefore account for GABA B receptor deficits. The specificity of these changes, both in terms of receptor subtype and anatomical localization may explain why a previous study using a tissue homogenate preparation of temporal cortex and [^{3}H]-muscimol, which does not differentiate A and B type receptors, failed to find any alteration in total GABA receptors[124]. Alternatively a more severe loss of neuronal elements in temporal cortex as compared to frontal cortex may mask any receptor deficit in the former. A 50% loss of total GABA receptor has been reported in homogenates of frontal cortex[170] while benzodiazepine receptors, which are linked to the GABA A receptor, were modestly reduced both in frontal cortex[171] and in temporal cortex[124,171].

A presynaptic location on cholinergic afferents may explain, at least in part, the reduction in cortical somatostatin receptors[172] as these receptors are also reduced following experimental lesions of the basal forebrain[173]. In contrast, to these receptor deficits there is a reciprocal increase in cortical CRF receptors associated with a local loss of this peptide[164] which suggests that whatever elements these receptors are localized on they are capable of CRF receptor upregulation in response to a loss of input.

Functional capability of neurotransmitter receptors in Alzheimer's disease

While a variety of neurotransmitter receptors are lost in Alzheimer's disease, it is obvious that there are a number of different receptors which are preserved or even increased in number. Receptors may be present on the membranes of neurones whose intracellular functions are disrupted, e.g. by the presence of tangles. Moreover, the persistence of a receptor recognition site does not necessarily imply that it retains its physiological integrity. In other words, while radioligand binding assays detect the binding of a neuro-transmitter analogue to a specific receptor recognition site, this does not mean that in vivo such an event would result in a functional response. The presence of muscarinic receptors within plaques[99] implies that these receptors are not involved in the mediation of normal neuronal activity.

Cellular responses to neurotransmitter receptor activation depend on the integrity of the coupling of the receptor recognition sites to their associated signal transduction mechanisms. Activation of a receptor results in its coupling to a guanine nucleotide binding protein (G protein) and this in turn, activates or inhibits associated second messenger systems. The two major second messenger systems in brain are generation of cyclic AMP by the enzyme adenylate cyclase or the phosphoinositide cycle, whereby hydrolysis of membrane lipids activates certain phosphorylating enzymes and mobilizes intracellular calcium[174,175]. Assessment of these second messenger systems can therefore provide an indication of the functional capabilities of their associated receptors. Radiolabelled ligands which bind to components within these two systems provide useful tools for the investigation of second messenger systems in post-mortem brain tissue.

Adenylate cyclase system

A variety of different receptor types are linked to the adenylate cyclase system and receptor activation either stimulates or inhibits adenylate cyclase depending on the particular receptor involved. Receptors which stimulate adenylate cyclase activity include β-adrenergic, dopamine (D_1), adenosine A_2, $5HT_1$ and VIP receptors while those that inhibit this enzyme include α_2 adrenergic, adenosine A_1, GABA B, M_2 muscarinic and opiate (u) receptors[174].

The stimulatory arm of the adenylate cyclase system has been investigated in Alzheimer brain by means of quantitative [^{3}H]-forskolin binding auto-radiography. [^{3}H]-forskolin binds to sites which are thought to be associated with the stimulatory G protein (Gs) linked to adenylate cyclase[176]. In Alzheimer brains, in which there were substantial reductions in ChAT

79

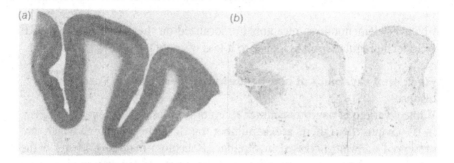

Fig. 6. Representative autoradiograms generated by incubating sections of human brain with 20 nM [³H]-forskolin which labels the stimulatory arm of the adenylate cyclase second messenger system. (a) and (b) are sections of middle frontal gyrus from (a) control and (b) an AD case. From Dewar et al[177].

activity and numerous plaques, in frontal and temporal cortices and the hippocampus, [³H]-forskolin binding sites were not uniformly altered within the same three brain regions[177]. [³H]-forskolin binding was markedly reduced throughout all layers of frontal cortex in Alzheimer cases compared to controls (Fig. 6). In contrast to the frontal cortex, in the hippocampal region, there was no alteration in the level of [³H]-forskolin binding and in the same group of patients there was an inconsistent reduction in the amount of [³H]-forskolin binding in the temporal cortex although ChAT activity was significantly reduced in all cases and the mean number of plaques in this brain region was similar to that observed in frontal cortex. It was noted that only some of the patients had significantly reduced [³H]-forskolin binding in temporal cortex while all Alzheimer patients had reduced [³H]-forskolin binding in frontal cortex. These differences between brain areas and between patients may be attributed to differences in the degree of neuronal fallout. However, preservation of [³H]-forskolin binding in hippocampus and, in some patients, in temporal cortex does not support this. Neuronal loss in CA1 of the hippocampus can be up to 50% of control values[104], whereas [³H]-forskolin binding remained unaltered. Moreover, neuronal loss from middle temporal cortex is reported to be of similar magnitude to that observed in frontal cortex.

There is strong evidence to suggest that high affinity [³H]-forskolin binding sites are associated with the Gs binding protein[176]. Receptors which stimulate adenylate cyclase through Gs include β-adrenergic, dopamine D_1, serotonergic, adenosine A_2, and VIP receptors. Reductions of $5HT_1$ receptors in frontal cortex have been reported in Alzheimer brains[29,121], although the deficit was only approximately 25% of controls. These losses could account for some of the [³H]-forskolin binding deficit. Neither B_1 nor B_2 adrenoreceptors were reduced in frontal cortex[133] and B_2 receptors were increased in this brain region[134]. Thus, it could be inferred that while a majority of recognition sites are preserved, or even increased, there is a significant loss of their associated G proteins, Gs. Of the other receptors which are linked to Gs, it is unclear whether their numbers are altered in Alzheimer patients. Total dopamine receptors (D_1 and D_2) as measured by [^{3}H]-spiroperidol binding are not reduced in frontal cortex[170], but no information about adenosine A_2 or VIP receptors exists. A loss of elements containing these receptors may contribute to the [^{3}H]-forskolin binding deficit but this remains to be established. Possible explanations for these findings include a selective loss of the elements to which forskolin binds in frontal cortex. Or that in the hippocampus and in some cases in the middle temporal gyrus, compensatory mechanisms have come into play to upregulate these elements in response to receptor loss. In regard to a possible upregulation of the adenylate cyclase system in Alzheimer's disease, Danielsson et al[178] reported elevated adenylate cyclase activity in the hippocampus. However, the amount of enzyme activity stimulated by activation of VIP receptors was no different in Alzheimer brains compared to controls. In the parietal cortex there was no alteration in adenylate cyclase activity in Alzheimer patients.

Phosphoinositide system

The phosphoinositide cycle has received slightly more attention than the adenylate cyclase system in post-mortem studies of Alzheimer brain, most probably because it is associated with muscarinic cholinergic receptors. This system also mediates the actions of neurotransmitters at $5HT_2$, α_1-adrenergic, a number of peptide receptors[175] as well as some excitatory amino acid receptors[179]. A full description of the way in which this second messenger system operates can be found in a number of excellent reviews[175,180]. Briefly, the binding of a transmitter to its receptor activates the associated G protein which in turn stimulates the enzyme phospholipase C to hydrolyse phosphatidylinositol 4,5-*bis*-phosphate (PIP_2). This reaction generates both inositol 1,4,5-triphosphate (IP_3) and diacylglycerol. IP_3 binds to a receptor located on the endoplasmic reticulum bringing about a release of intracellular Ca^{2+}. Diacylglycerol activates protein kinase C (PKC) which phosphorylates a wide range of substances. The manufacture of [^{3}H]-IP_3 and [^{3}H]-phorbol esters (which bind to PKC) means that useful tools are available for investigation of this system in post mortem brain.

The coupling of muscarinic M_1 receptors to their associated G protein was found to be altered in the parietal cortex in Alzheimer brain although the authors do not exclude the possibility that differences in the agonal status of Alzheimer and control subjects may have influenced the results[181]. Experiments in rats, which have received lesions of the ascending cholinergic projection from the basal forebrain, suggest that the phosphoinositide second messenger system linked to muscarinic receptors is unaltered in the long-term, by such treatment[182]. Although a large increase in carbachol-stimulated phosphoinositide hydrolysis was observed 5 days following the cholinergic lesion, their response was no different from unlesioned animals at 50 and 118 days post lesion[183]. These results suggest that cholinergic denervation alone does not alter the functional capability of muscarinic receptors. In the temporal cortex of Alzheimer brain, a reduction in the level of PIP_2 was found while the levels of other polyphosphoinositides were unchanged[184]. A comprehensive study of 7 different regions of Alzheimer brain revealed severe losses (50–70%) of $[^3H]$-IP_3 binding in parietal cortex and hippocampus. Although there appeared to be some degree of loss from other cortical areas (particularly frontal cortex) and the amygdala, compared to controls these did not reach statistical significance[185].

The amount of PKC, as measured both by $[^3H]$-phorbol ester binding levels or enzyme activity in frontal cortex was 50% less in Alzheimer than in control subjects[186]. Moreover, the phosphorylation of an endogenous substrate by PKC also was reduced in Alzheimer frontal cortex although reduced levels of phosphorylation were observed in demented patients who had Pick's disease. Severe neuronal degeneration is a feature of Pick's disease and therefore it was suggested that the reduced PKC levels and activity were not solely due to neuronal fallout in the Alzheimer cases. Cole and colleagues[186] also point out that PKC is involved in the survival and maintenance of neurones and thus a loss of PKC activity in Alzheimer's disease may have important implications for neuronal degeneration.

What is unclear in these studies of second messenger systems in Alzheimer's disease is to what degree a loss of their markers represents the effects of non-selective neuronal degeneration. It would be interesting to know the extent to which other markers (e.g. for specific receptors linked to a particular system) are altered or preserved within the same sample of brain tissue. Simultaneous assessment of multiple receptor recognition sites and post-receptor systems may shed light on whether receptor recognition sites are altered before, after or at the same time as second messenger systems. Asynchronous alterations of these two components will have obvious implications for any therapeutic strategies aimed at treatment of Alzheimer's disease. The possibility of second messenger systems as targets for therapeutic intervention remains to be investigated experimentally.

Conclusion

Many studies of the neurotransmitter deficits in Alzheimer's disease appear to have been directed by the possibility of replacement therapy; particularly with regard to the cholinergic system. After more than a decade of research, however, it is clear that, at least at post-mortem there are a multitude of neurotransmitter and receptor abnormalities. The question posed in most studies appears to be: is there a change in a particular variable in Alzheimer brains compared to controls? However, a more appropriately framed question may be: if a particular neurochemical variable changes, how does this relate to, on the one hand, the underlying *local* structural changes and on the other, changes in other related neurochemical parameters, within the same tissue sample. Neurotransmitter and receptor abnormalities may precede, accompany or respond to local structural degeneration and more valuable insight regarding the temporal relationships between the morphological degenerative processes of the disease and neurochemical abnormalities may be gained if more correlative analyses within the same patients are undertaken, in future.

Although Alzheimer's disease is a neurodegenerative condition, there is some evidence which suggests that, at least some neurotransmitter systems have a capacity for plastic, possibly compensatory change. This is illustrated by the number of studies which report an increase in the level of neurotransmitter receptors including glutamate[78,92], muscarinic[104], β-adrenergic[130,134] and CRF[164] receptors. The phenomenon of receptor supersensitivity, in response to a loss of presynaptic input, is well known and this may apply, in some instances, in the Alzheimer brain. However, the occurrence of this phenomenon may be complicated by concomitant post-synaptic degeneration. Indeed, these two events may explain why there are many studies which report no change in receptor levels. Moreover, the possibility of a threshold of neuronal loss beyond which compensatory mechanisms involved in receptor regulation are unable to function should be considered[104].

The outlook for any form of transmitter replacement therapy for Alzheimer's disease must be extremely pessimistic, in view of the multifarious nature of the transmitter and receptor changes which occur in this condition. In addition, although in some instances neurotransmitter receptors appear to be preserved, abnormalities in their associated second messenger systems may render such receptors functionally useless. However, an understanding of the mechanisms by which neurones attempt to maintain synaptic transmission, whether in response to presynaptic loss or to local morphological change, may provide crucial information regarding both the degenerative process of Alzheimer's disease and possible avenues of therapeutic intervention.

Acknowledgements
We are grateful to our colleagues, Ms Karen Horsburgh and Professor David Graham, for their invaluable contributions to the work from the Wellcome Neuroscience Group, Glasgow, described in this chapter. This work was entirely supported by the Wellcome Trust. We would also like to thank Ann Marie Colquhoun for her excellent secretarial assistance in the preparation of the manuscript.

D Dewar

References

(1) Terry RD, Peck A, DeTeresa R, Schechter R, Horoupian DS. Some morphometric aspects of the brain in senile dementia of the Alzheimer type. *Ann Neurol* 1981; 10: 184–92.

(2) Davies P, Maloney AFJ. Selective loss of cerebral cholinergic neurones in Alzheimer's disease. *Lancet* 1976; ii: 1403.

(3) Bowen DM, Smith CB, White P, Davison AN. Neurotransmitter related enzymes and indices of hypoxia in senile dementia and other abiotrophies. *Brain* 1976; 99: 459–96.

(4) Perry EK, Perry RH, Blessed G, Tomlinson BE. Necropsy evidence of cerebral cholinergic deficits in senile dementia. *Lancet* 1977; i: 1–89.

(5) Höhmann C, Antuono P, Coyle JT. Basal forebrain cholinergic neurons and Alzheimer's disease. In: Iversen LL, Iversen SD, Snyder SH, eds. *Handbook of Psychopharmacology*. New York: Plenum Press, 1988; 20: 69–106.

(6) Hedreen JC, Struble RG, Whitehouse PJ, Price DL. Topography of the magnocellular basal forebrain system in human brain. *J Neuropathol Exp Neurol* 1984; 43: 1–21.

(7) Arendt T, Bigl V, Arendt A, Tennstedt A. Loss of neurones in nucleus basalis of Meynert in Alzheimer's disease, paralysis agitans and Korsakoff's disease. *Acta Neuropathol* 1983; 61: 101–8.

(8) Arendt T, Bigl V, Tennstedt A, Arendt A. Neuronal loss in different parts of the nucleus basalis is related to neuritic plaque formation in cortical target areas in Alzheimer's disease. *Neuroscience* 1985; 14: 1–14.

(9) Tagliavini F, Pilleri G. Basal nucleus of Meynert. *J Neurol Sci* 1983; 62: 243–60.

(10) Whitehouse PJ, Price DL, Strubel RG, Clark AW, Coyle JT, Delong MR. Alzheimer's disease and senile dementia. Loss of neurones in the basal forebrain. *Science* 1982; 215: 1237–9.

(11) Perry EK, Tomlinson BE, Blessed G, Bergmann K, Gibson PH, Perry RH. Correlation of cholinergic abnormalities with senile plaques and mental test scores in senile dementia. *Br Med J* 1978; 2: 1457–9.

(12) Sahakian BJ. Cholinergic drugs and human cognitive performance. In: Iversen LL, Iversen SD, Snyder SH, eds. *Handbook of Psychopharmacology*. New York: Plenum Press, 1988: 393–424.

(13) Hagan JJ, Morris RGM. The cholinergic hypothesis of memory: a review of animal experiments. In: Iversen LL, Iversen SD, Snyder SH, eds. *Handbook of Psychopharmacology*. New York: Plenum Press, 1988: 237–323.

(14) Wilcock GK, Esiri MM, Bowen DM, Hughes AO. The differential involvement of subcortical nuclei in senile dementia of Alzheimer's type. *J Neurol Neurosurg Psychiat* 1988; 51: 842–9.

(15) Etienne P, Robitaille Y, Wood P, Gauthier S, Nair NPV, Quirion R. Nucleus basalis neuronal loss, neuritic plaques and choline acetyltransferase activity in advanced Alzheimer's disease. *Neuroscience* 1986; 19: 1279–91.

(16) Pearson RCH, Sofronie MV, Cuello AC et al. Persistence of cholinergic neurons in the basal nucleus in a brain with senile dementia of Alzheimer type demonstrated by immunohistochemical staining for choline acetyltransferase. *Brain Res* 1983; 289: 375–9.

(17) Mesulam M-M. Alzheimer plaques and cortical cholinergic innervation. *Neuroscience* 1986; 17: 275–6.

(18) Arendt T, Bigl V. Alzheimer plaques and cortical cholinergic innervation. *Neuroscience* 1986; 17: 277–9.

(19) Masliah E, Terry R, Buzsaki G. Thalamic nuclei in Alzheimer disease: evidence against the cholinergic hypothesis of plaque formation. *Brain Res* 1989; 493: 240–6.

(20) Kitt CA, Price DL, Strubel RG et al. Evidence for cholinergic neurites in senile plaques. *Science* 1984; 226: 1443–4.

(21) Armstrong DM, Bruce G, Hersh LB, Terry RD. Choline acetyltransferase immunoreactivity in neuritic plaques of Alzheimer's brain. *Neurosci Lett* 1986; 71: 229–34.

(22) Walker LC, Kitt CA, Struble RG et al. Glutamic acid decarboxylase like immunoreactive neurites in senile plaques. *Neurosci Lett* 1985; 59: 165–9.

(23) Chan-Palay V, Lang W, Allen YS, Haesler U, Polak JM. II. Cortical neurons immunoreactive with antisera against neuropeptide Y are altered in Alzheimer type dementia. *J Comp Neurol* 1985; 238: 390–400.

(24) Armstrong DM, Benzing WC, Evans J, Terry RD, Shields D, Hansen LA. Substance P and somatostatin coexist within neuritic plaques: implications for the pathogenesis of Alzheimer's disease. *Neuroscience* 1989; 31: 663–71.

(25) Struble RG, Powers RE, Casanova MF, Kitt CA, Brown EC, Price DL. Neuropeptide systems in plaques of Alzheimer's disease. *J Neuropath exp. Neurol* 1987; 46: 567–84.

(26) Armstrong DM, Terry RD. Substance P immunoreactivity within neuritic plaques. *Neurosci Lett* 1985; 58: 139–44.

(27) Cross AJ, Crow TJ, Johnson JA et al. Monoamine metabolism in senile dementia of Alzheimer type. *J Neurol Sci* 1983; 60: 383–92.

(28) Arai H, Kosaka K, Iizuka R. Changes of biogenic amines and their metabolites in post mortem brain from patients with Alzheimer type dementia. *J Neurochem* 1984; 43: 388–93.

(29) Bowen DM, Allen SJ, Benton JS. Biochemical assessment of serotonergic and cholinergic dysfunction and cerebral atrophy in Alzheimer's disease. *J Neurochem* 1983; 41: 266–72.

(30) Burke WJ, Chung HD, Huang JS et al. Evidence for retrograde degeneration of epinephrine neurons in Alzheimer's disease. *Ann Neurol* 1988; 24: 532–6.

(31) Herregodts P, Bruyland M, De Keyser J, Solheid C, Michotte Y, Ebinger G. Monoaminergic neurotransmitters in Alzheimer's disease. An HPLC study comparing presenile familial and sporadic senile cases. *J Neurol Sci* 1989; 92: 101–16.

(32) Baker GB, Reynolds GP. Biogenic amines and their metabolites in Alzheimer's disease: noradrenaline, 5-hydroxytryptamine and 5-hydroxyindole-3-acetic acid depleted in hippocampus but not in substantia innominata. *Neurosci Lett* 1989; 335–9.

(33) Tomlinson BE, Irving D, Blessed G. Cell loss in the locus caeruleus in senile dementia of Alzheimer's type. *J Neurol Sci* 1981; 49: 419–28.

(34) Bondareff W, Mountjoy CQ, Roth M. Selective loss of neurons of origin of

adrenergic projection to cerebral cortex (nucleus locus caeruleus) in senile dementia. *Lancet* 1981; i: 783–4.

(35) Yamamoto T, Hirano A. Nucleus raphe dorsalis in Alzheimer's disease: neuro-fibrillary tangles and loss of large neurons. *Ann Neurol* 1985; 17: 573–7.

(36) Mann DMA, Yates PO, Marcyniuk B. Monoaminergic neurotransmitter systems in presenile Alzheimer's Disease and in senile dementia of Alzheimer type. *Clin Neuropathol* 1984; 3: 199–205.

(37) Chan-Palay V, Asan E. Alterations in catecholamine neurons of locus coeruleus in senile dementia of the Alzheimer type and in Parkinson's disease with and without dementia and depression. *J Comp Neurol* 1989; 287: 373–92.

(38) Sims NR, Bowen DM, Allen SJ et al. Presynaptic cholinergic dysfunction in patients with dementia. *J Neurochem* 1983; 40: 503–9.

(39) Perry EK, Curtis M, Dick DJ et al. Cholinergic correlates of cognitive impairment in Parkinson's disease: comparisons with Alzheimer's disease. *J Neurol Neurosurg Psychiatry* 1985; 48: 413–21.

(40) Cross AJ, Slater P, Simpson M et al. Sodium dependent [^{3}H]-d-aspartate binding in cerebral cortex in patients with Alzheimer's and Parkinson's diseases. *Neurosci Lett* 1987; 79: 213–17.

(41) Kish SJ, El-Awar M, Schut L, Leach L, Oscar-Berman M, Freedman M. Cognitive deficits in olivopontocerebellar atropy: implications for the cholinergic hypothesis of Alzheimer's dementia. *Ann Neurol* 1988; 24: 200–6.

(42) Kish SJ, Schut L, Simmons J, Gilbert J, Chang L-J, Rebbetoy M. Brain acetylcholinesterase activity is markedly reduced in dominantly-inherited olivopontocerebellar atrophy. *J Neurol Neurosurg Psychiatry* 1988; 51: 544–8.

(43) Wood PL, Etienne P, Lal S et al. A post-mortem comparison of the cortical cholinergic system in Alzheimer's disease and Pick's disease. *J Neurol Sci* 1983; 62: 211–17.

(44) Uhl GR, Hilt DC, Hedreen JC, Whitehouse PJ, Price DL. Pick's disease (lobar sclerosis): Depletion of neurons in the nucleus basalis of Meynert. *Neurology* 1983; 33: 1470–3.

(45) Neary D, Snowden JS, Mann DMA et al. Alzheimer's disease: a correlative study. *J Neurol Neurosurg Psychiatry* 1986; 49: 229–37.

(46) Rogers J, Morrison JH. Quantitative morphology and regional and laminar distributions of senile plaques in Alzheimer's disease. *J Neurosci* 1985; 5: 2801–8.

(47) Pearson RCA, Esiri MM, Hiorns RW, Wilocock GK, Powell TPS. Anatomical correlates of the distribution of the pathological changes in the neocortex in Alzheimer's disease. *Proc Natl Acad Sci USA* 1985; 82: 4531–4.

(48) Terry RD, Katzman R. Senile dementia of Alzheimer's type. *Ann Neurol* 1983; 14: 497–506.

(49) Kemper T. Neuroanatomical and neuropathological changes in normal aging and in dementia. In: Albert ML, ed. *Clinical Neurology of Aging*. New York: Oxford University Press, 1984: 9–52.

(50) Tomlinson BE, Blessed G, Roth M. Observations on the brains of non-demented old people. *J Neurol Sci* 1968; 7: 331–56.

(51) Tomlinson BE, Blessed G, Roth M. Observations on the brains of demented old people. *J Neurol Sci* 1970; 11: 205–42.

(52) Duyckaerts C, Hauw J-J, Bastenaire F et al. Laminar distribution of neocortical

plaques in senile dementia of the Alzheimer type. *Acta Neuropathol* 1986; 70: 249–56.

(53) Lewis DA, Campbell MJ, Terry RD, Morrison JH. Laminar and regional distributions of neurofibrillary tangles and neuritic plaques in Alzheimer's disease: A quantitative study of visual and auditory cortices. *J Neurosci* 1987; 7: 1799–808.

(54) Mountjoy CQ, Roth M, Evans NJR, Evans HM. Cortical neuronal counts in normal elderly controls and demented patients. *Neurobiol Aging* 1983; 4: 1–11.

(55) Hubbard BM, Anderson JM. Age-related variations in the neuron content of the cerebral cortex in senile dementia of Alzheimer type. *Neuropath Appl Neurobiol* 1985; 11: 369–82.

(56) Mann DMA, Yates PO, Marcyniuk B. Some morphometric observations on the cerebral cortex and hippocampus in presenile Alzheimer's disease, senile dementia of Alzheimer type and Down's syndrome in middle age. *J Neurol Sci* 1985; 69: 139–59.

(57) Davies CA, Mann DMA, Sumpter PQ, Yates PO. A quantitative morphometric analysis of the neuronal and synaptic content of the frontal and temporal cortex in patients with Alzheimer's disease. *J Neurol Sci* 1987; 78: 151–64.

(58) Fonnum F, Soreide A, Kvale I, Walker J, Walaas I. Glutamate in cortical fibers. *Adv Biochem Psychopharmacol* 1981; 27: 29–41.

(59) Emson PC, Lindvall O. Neuroanatomical aspects of neurotransmitters affected in Alzheimer's Disease. *British Medical Bulletin* 1986; 42: 57–62.

(60) Shank RP, Campbell GleM. Glutamate. In: Lajtha A, ed. *Handbook of Neurochemistry*. New York: Plenum Press, 1983; 3: 381–404.

(61) Arai H, Kobayashi K, Ichimiya Y, Kosaka K, Iizuka R. Free amino acids in post-mortem cerebral cortices from patients with Alzheimer-type dementia. *Neurosci Res* 1985; 2: 486–90.

(62) Sasaki H, Muramoto O, Kanazawa I, Arai H, Kosaka K, Iizuka R. Regional distribution of amino acid transmitters in postmortem brains of presenile and senile dementia of Alzheimer type. *Ann Neurol* 1986; 19: 263–9.

(63) Ellison DW, Beal MF, Mazurek MF, Bird ED, Martin JB. A postmortem study of amino acid neurotransmitters in Alzheimer's disease. *Ann Neurol* 1986; 20: 616–21.

(64) Hyman BT, Van Hoesen GW, Damasio AR. Alzheimer's disease: glutamate depletion in the hippocampal perforant pathway zone. *Ann Neurol* 1987; 22: 37–40.

(65) Procter AW, Palmer AM, Francis PT et al. Evidence of glutamatergic denervation and possible abnormal metabolism in Alzheimer's disease. *J Neurochem* 1988; 50: 790–802.

(66) Tarbit I, Perry EK, Perry RH, Blessed G, Tomlinson BE. Hippocampal free amino acids in Alzheimer's disease. *J Neurochem* 1980; 35: 1246–9.

(67) Perry TL, Yong VW, Bergeron C, Hansen S, Jones K. Amino acids, glutathione, and glutathione transferase activity in the brains of patients with Alzheimer's disease. *Ann Neurol* 1987; 21: 331–6.

(68) Smith CCT, Bowen DM, Sims NR, Neary D, Davison AN. Amino acid release from biopsy samples of temporal neocortex from patients with Alzheimer's disease. *Brain Res* 1983; 264: 138–41.

(69) Cross AJ, Skan WJ, Slater P. The association of [^{3}H]D-aspartate binding and

high affinity glutamate uptake in the human brain. *Neurosci Lett* 1986; 63: 121–4.

(70) Procter AW, Palmer AM, Stratmann GC, Bowen DM. Glutamate/Aspartate-releasing neurons in Alzheimer's disease. *N Eng J Med* 1986; 314: 1711–12.

(71) Palmer AM, Procter AW, Stratmann GC, Bowen DM. Excitatory amino acid-releasing and cholinergic neurones in Alzheimer's disease. *Neurosci Lett* 1986; 66: 199–204.

(72) Cross AJ, Slater P, Candy JM, Perry EK, Perry RH. Glutamate deficits in Alzheimer's disease. *J Neurol Neurosurg Psychiat* 1987; 50: 357–8.

(73) Simpson MDC, Royston MC, Deakin JFW, Cross AJ, Mann DMA, Slater P. Regional changes in $[^3H]$-d-aspartate and $[^3H]$-TCP binding sites in Alzheimer's disease brains. *Brain Res* 1988; 462: 76–82.

(74) Cowburn R, Hardy J, Roberts P, Briggs R. Regional distribution of pre- and postsynaptic glutamatergic function in Alzheimer's disease. *Brain Res* 1988; 452: 403–7.

(75) Cowburn R, Hardy J, Roberts P, Briggs R. Presynaptic and postsynaptic glutamatergic function in Alzheimer's disease. *Neurosci Lett* 1988; 86: 109–13.

(76) Hardy J, Cowburn R, Barton A et al. Region-specific loss of glutamate innervation in Alzheimer's disease. *Neurosci Lett* 1987; 73: 77–80.

(77) Procter AW, Lowe SL, Palmer AM et al. Topographical distribution of neurochemical changes in Alzheimer's disease. *J Neurol Sci* 1988; 84: 125–40.

(78) Chalmers DT, Dewar D, Graham DI, Brooks DN, McCulloch J. Differential alterations of cortical glutamatergic binding sites in senile dementia of the Alzheimer type. *Proc Natl Acad Sci USA* 1990; 87: 1352–6.

(79) Charlton FG, Candy JM, Perry EK, Perry RH. The status of excitatory dicarboxylic amino acid uptake sites in the cerebral cortex in Alzheimer's and Parkinson's diseases. *Br J Pharmacol* 1989; 96: 350P.

(80) Watkins JC, Krogsgaard-Larsen P, Honore T. Structure–activity relationships in the development of excitatory amino acid receptor agonists and competitive antagonists. *Trends Pharmacol Sci* 1990; 11: 25–33.

(81) Morris RGM, Anderson E, Lynch G, Baudry M. Selective impairment of learning and blockade of long term potentiation by an N-methyl-d-aspartate receptor antagonist, AP-5. *Nature* 1986; 319: 774–6.

(82) Greenamyre JT, Penney JB, Young AB, D'Amato CJ, Hicks SP, Shoulson I. Alterations in L-glutamate binding in Alzheimer's and Huntington's diseases. *Science* 1985; 227: 1496–9.

(83) Hardy J, Cowburn R. Glutamate neurotoxicity and Alzheimer's disease. *Trends Neurosci* 1987; 10: 406.

(84) Maragos WF, Greenamyre JT, Penney JB, Young AB. Reply from W. F. Maragos and colleagues. *Trends Neurosci* 1987; 10: 407.

(85) Mouradian MM, Contreras PC, Monahan JB, Chase TN. $[^3H]$-MK-801 binding in Alzheimer's disease. *Neurosci Lett* 1988; 93: 225–30.

(86) Geddes JW, Chang-Chui H, Cooper SM, Lott IT, Cotman CW. Density and distribution of NMDA receptors in the human hippocampus in Alzheimer's disease. *Brain Res* 1986; 399: 156–61.

(87) Monaghan DT, Geddes JW, Yao D, Chung C, Cotman W. $[^3H]$-TCP binding sites in Alzheimer's disease. *Neurosci Lett* 1987; 73: 197–200.

(88) Greenamyre JT, Penney JB, D'Amato CJ, Young AB. Dementia of the Alzheimer's type: changes in hippocampal L-[^{3}H]-glutamate binding. *J Neurochem* 1987; 48: 543–51.

(89) Maragos WF, Chu DCM, Young AB, D'Amato CJ, Penney JB. Loss of hippocampal [^{3}H]-TCP binding in Alzheimer's disease. *Neurosci Lett* 1987; 74: 371–6.

(90) Represa A, Duyckaerts C, Tremblay E, Hauw JJ, Ben-Ari Y. Is senile dementia of the Alzheimer type associated with hippocampal plasticity? *Brain Res* 1988; 457: 355–9.

(91) Cowburn RF, Hardy JA, Briggs RS, Roberts PJ. Characterisation, density, and distribution of kainate receptors in normal and Alzheimer's diseased human brain. *J Neurochem* 1989; 52: 140–7.

(92) Geddes JW, Monaghan DT, Cotman CW, Lott IT, Kim RC, Chui HC. Plasticity of hippocampal circuitry in Alzheimer's disease. *Science* 1985; 230: 1179–81.

(93) Pearce BR, Bowen DM. [^{3}H]-Kainic acid binding and choline acetyltransferase activity in Alzheimer's dementia. *Brain Res* 1984; 310: 376–8.

(94) Maragos WF, Greenamyre JT, Penney JB, Young AB. Glutamate dysfunction in Alzheimer's disease: an hypothesis. *Trends Neurosci* 1987; 10: 65–8.

(95) Collingridge GL. Long term potentiation in the hippocampus: mechanisms of initiation and modulation by neurotransmitters. *Trends Pharmacol Sci* 1985; 6: 407–11.

(96) Rothman SM, Olney JW. Excitotoxicity and the NMDA receptor. *Trends Neurosci* 1987; 10: 299–302.

(97) Sofroniew MV, Pearson RCA. Degeneration of cholinergic neurons in the basal nucleus following kainic or N-methyl-D-aspartic acid application to the cerebral cortex in the rat. *Brain Res* 1985; 339: 186–90.

(98) Caulfield MP, Straughan DW, Cross AJ, Crow T, Birdsall NJ. Cortical muscarinic receptor subtypes and Alzheimer's disease. *Lancet* 1982; ii: 1277.

(99) Palacios JM. Autoradiographic localization of muscarinic cholinergic receptors in the hippocampus of patients with senile dementia. *Brain Res* 1982; 23: 173–5.

(100) Mash DC, Flynn DD, Potter LT. Loss of M2 muscarine receptors in the cerebral cortex in Alzheimer's disease and experimental cholinergic denervation. *Science* 1985; 228: 1115–17.

(101) Araujo DM, Lapchak PA, Robitaille Y, Gauthier S, Quirion R. Differential alteration of various cholinergic markers in cortical and subcortical regions of human brain in Alzheimer's disease. *J Neurochem* 1988; 50: 1914–23.

(102) Smith CJ, Perry EK, Perry RH et al. Muscarinic cholinergic receptor subtypes in hippocampus in human cognitive disorders. *J Neurochem* 1988; 50: 847–56.

(103) Rinne JO, Lönnberg P, Marjamäki P, Rinne UK. Brain muscarinic receptor subtypes are differently affected in Alzheimer's disease and Parkinson's disease. *Brain Res* 1989; 483: 402–6.

(104) Probst A, Cortes R, Ulrich J, Palacios JM. Differential modification of muscarinic cholinergic receptors in the hippocampus of patients with Alzheimer's disease: an autoradiographic study. *Brain Res* 1988; 450: 190–201.

(105) Shimohama S, Taniguchi T, Fujiwara M, Kameyama M. Changes in nicotinic

and muscarinic cholinergic receptors in Alzheimer-type dementia. *J Neurochem* 1986; 46: 288–93.

(106) Lang W, Henke H. Cholinergic receptor binding and autoradiography in brains of non-neurological and senile dementia of Alzheimer-type patients. *Brain Res* 1983; 267: 271–80.

(107) Waller SB, Ball MJ, Reynolds MA, London ED. Muscarinic binding and choline acetyltransferase in postmortem brains of demented patients. *Can J Neurol Sci* 1986; 13: 528–32.

(108) Ruberg M, Ploska A, Javoy-Agid F, Agid Y. Muscarinic binding and choline acetyl transferase activity in Parkinsonian subjects with reference to dementia. *Brain Res* 1982; 232: 129–39.

(109) Perry EK, Perry RH, Smith CJ et al. Cholinergic receptors in cognitive disorders. *Can J Neurol Sci* 1986; 13: 521–7.

(110) de Belleroche J, Gardiner IM, Hamilton MH, Birdsall NJM. Analysis of muscarinic receptor concentration and subtypes following lesion of rat substantia innominata. *Brain Res* 1985; 340: 201–9.

(111) Atack JR, Wenk GL, Wagster MV, Kellar KJ, Whitehouse PJ, Rapoport SI. Bilateral changes in neocortical [^{3}H]-pirenzepine and [^{3}H]-oxotremorine-M binding following unilateral lesions of the rat nucleus basalis magnocellularis: an autoradiographic study. *Brain Res* 1989; 483: 367–72.

(112) Nordberg A, Winblad B. Reduced number of [^{3}H]-nicotine and [^{3}H]-acetylcholine binding sites in the frontal cortex of Alzheimer brains. *Neurosci Lett* 1986; 72: 115–19.

(113) Nordberg A, Adem A, Hardy J, Winblad B. Change in nicotinic receptor subtypes in temporal cortex of Alzheimer brains. *Neurosci Lett* 1988; 86: 317–21.

(114) Whitehouse PJ, Martino AM, Antuono PG et al. Nicotinic acetylcholine binding sites in Alzheimer's disease. *Brain Res* 1986; 371: 146–51.

(115) Whitehouse PJ, Kellar KJ. Nicotinic and muscarinic cholinergic receptors in Alzheimer's disease and related disorders. *J Neural Transm* 1987; 24: 175–82.

(116) Whitehouse PJ, Martino AM, Wagster MV et al. Reductions in [^{3}H]-nicotinic acetylcholine binding in Alzheimer's disease and Parkinson's disease: An autoradiographic study. *Neurology* 1988; 38: 720–3.

(117) Perry EK, Perry RH, Smith CJ et al. Nicotinic receptor abnormalities in Alzheimer's and Parkinson's disease. *J Neurol Neurosurg Psychiat* 1987; 50: 806–9.

(118) Rowell PP, Winkler DL. Nicotinic stimulation of [^{3}H]-acetylcholine release from mouse cerebral cortical synaptosomes. *J Neurochem* 1984; 43: 1593–8.

(119) Schwartz RD, Lehmann J, Kellar KJ. Presynaptic nicotinic cholinergic receptors labeled by [^{3}H]acetylcholine on catecholamine and serotonin axons in brain. *J Neurochem* 1984; 42: 1495–8.

(120) Morrow AL, Loy R, Creese I. Alterations of nicotinic cholinergic agonist binding sites in hippocampus after fimbria transection. *Brain Res* 1985; 334: 309–14.

(121) Cross AJ, Crow TJ, Johnson JA et al. Studies of neurotransmitter receptor systems in neocortex and hippocampus in senile dementia of the Alzheimer-type. *J Neurol Sci* 1984; 64: 109–17.

(122) Reynolds GP, Arnold L, Rossor MN, Iversen Ll, Mountjoy CQ, Roth M.

Reduced binding of [^{3}H]-ketanserin to cortical 5-HT$_2$ receptors in senile dementia of the Alzheimer type. *Neurosci Lett* 1984; 44: 47–51.

(123) Sparks DL. Aging and Alzheimer's disease. Altered cortical serotonergic binding. *Arch Neurol* 1989; 46: 138–40.

(124) Cross AJ, Crow TJ, Ferrier IN, Johnson JA. The selectivity of the reduction of serotonin S$_2$ receptors in Alzheimer-type dementia. *Neurobiol Aging* 1986; 7: 3–7.

(125) Perry EK, Perry RH, Candy JM et al. Cortical serotonin-S$_2$ receptor binding abnormalities in patients with Alzheimer's disease: comparisons with Parkinson's disease. *Neurosci Lett* 1984; 51: 353–7.

(126) Pazos A, Probst A, Palacios JM. Serotonin receptors in the human brain-IV. Autoradiographic mapping of serotonin-2 receptors. *Neuroscience* 1987; 21: 123–39.

(127) Cross AJ, Slater P, Perry EK, Perry RH. An autoradiographic analysis of serotonin receptors in human temporal cortex: changes in Alzheimer-type dementia. *Neurochem Internat* 1988; 13: 89–96.

(128) Dewar D, Graham DI, McCulloch J. 5HT$_2$ receptors in dementia of the Alzheimer type: an autoradiographic study of frontal cortex and hippocampus. *J Neural Transm* 1991; in press.

(129) Vogt BA, Van Hoesen GW, Vogt LJ, Crino PB. Four classes of Alzheimer's disease: Neocortical neuropathology and alterations in neurotransmitter receptor binding [Abstract]. *Soc for Neurosci* 1989; 15: 859.

(130) Middlemiss DN, Palmer AM, Edel N, Bowen DM. Binding of the novel serotonin agonist 8-hydroxy-2-(di-n-propylamino) tetralin in normal and Alzheimer brain. *J Neurochem* 1986; 46: 993–6.

(131) D'Amato RJ, Zweig RM, Whitehouse PJ et al. Aminergic systems in Alzheimer's disease and Parkinson's disease. *Ann Neurol* 1987; 22: 229–36.

(132) Shimohama S, Taniguchi T, Fujiwara M, Kameyama M. Biochemical characterization of α-adrenergic receptors in human brain and changes in Alzheimer-type dementia. *J Neurochem* 1986; 47: 1294–301.

(133) Shimohama S, Taniguchi T, Fujiwara M, Kameyama M. Changes in β-adrenergic receptor subtypes in Alzheimer-type dementia. *J Neurochem* 1987; 48: 1215–21.

(134) Kalaria RN, Andorn AC, Tabaton M, Whitehouse PJ, Harik SI, Unnerstall JR. Adrenergic receptors in aging and Alzheimer's disease: Increased B$_2$-receptors in prefrontal cortex and hippocampus. *J Neurochem* 1989; 53: 1772–81.

(135) Rossor MN, Garrett NH, Johnson AJ, Mountjoy CQ, Roth M, Iversen LL. A post-mortem study of the cholinergic and GABA systems in senile dementia. *Brain* 1982; 105: 313–30.

(136) Ellison DW, Beal MF, Mazurek MF, Bird ED, Martin JB. A post mortem study of amino acid neurotransmitters in Alzheimer's disease. *Ann Neurol* 1986; 20: 616–21.

(137) Sasaki H, Muramoto O, Manazawa I, Arai H, Kosaka K, Iizuka R. Regional distribution of amino acid transmitters in postmortem brains of presenile and senile dementia of Alzheimer type. *Ann Neurol* 1986; 19: 263–9.

(138) Davies P. Neurotransmitter-related enzymes in senile dementia of the Alzheimer type. *Brain Research* 1979; 171: 319–27.

(139) Monfort JC, Javoy-Agid F, Hauw JJ, Dubois B, Agid Y. Brain glutamate

D Dewar

severity index. *Brain* 1985; 108: 301–13.
(140) Reinikainen KJ, Paljärvi L, Huuskonen M, Soininen H, Laakso M, Riekkinen
PJ. A post-mortem study of noradrenergic, serotonergic and GABAergic
neurons in Alzheimer's disease. *J Neurol Sci* 1988; 84: 101–16.
(141) Perry EK, Atack JR, Perry RH et al. Intralaminar neurochemical distributions
in human midtemporal cortex: comparison between Alzheimer's disease and
the normal. *J Neurochem* 1984; 42: 1402–10.
(142) Hardy J, Cowburn R, Barton A et al. A disorder of cortical GABAergic innervation in Alzheimer's disease. *Neurosci Lett* 1987; 73: 192–6.
(143) Simpson MDC, Cross AJ, Slater P, Deakin JFW. Loss of cortical GABA uptake
sites in Alzheimer's disease. *J Neural Transm* 1988; 71: 219–26.
(144) Davies P, Katzman R, Terry RD. Reduced somatostatin-like immunoreactivity
in cerebral cortex from cases of Alzheimer's disease and Alzheimer senile
dementia. *Nature* 1980; 288: 279–80.
(145) Rossor MN, Emson PC, Mountjoy CQ, Roth M, Iversen LL. Reduced
amounts of immunoreactive somatostatin in the temporal cortex of senile
dementia of Alzheimer type. *Neurosci Lett* 1980; 20: 383–7.
(146) Beal MF, Mazurek MF, Svendsen CN, Bird ED, Martin JB (1986). Widespread reduction of somatostatin-like immunoreactivity in the cerebral cortex in
Alzheimer's disease. *Ann Neurol* 1986; 20: 489–95.
(147) Beal MF, Kowall NW, Mazurek MF. Neuropeptides in Alzheimer's disease. *J
Neural Transm* 1987; 24: 163–74.
(148) Chan-Palay V. Somatostatin immunoreactive neurons in the human hippocampus and cortex shown by immunogold/silver intensification on vibratome
sections: coexistence with neuropeptide Y neurons, and effects in Alzheimer-
type dementia. *J Comp Neurol* 1987; 260: 201–23.
(149) Hendry SHC, Jones EG, DeFelipe J, Schmechel D, Brandon C, Emson PC.
Neuropeptide-containing neurons of the cerebral cortex are also GABAergic.
Proc Natl Acad Sci USA 1984; 81: 6526–30.
(150) Roberts GW, Crow TJ, Polak JM. Location of neuronal tangles in somatostatin
neurons in Alzheimer's disease. *Nature* 1985; 314: 92–4.
(151) Morrison JH, Rogers J, Scherr S, Benoit R, Bloom FE. Somatostatin
immunoreactivity in neuritic plaques of Alzheimer's patients. *Nature* 1985; 314:
90–2.
(152) Smith CCT, Bowen DM, Sims NR, Neary D, Davidson AN. Amino acid
release from biopsy samples of temporal neocortex from patients with
Alzheimer's disease. *Brain Res* 1983; 264: 138–41.
(153) Francis PT, Bowen DM, Lowe SL, Neary D, Mann DMA, Snowden JS.
Somatostatin content and release measured in cerebral biopsies from demented
patients. *J Neurol Sci* 1987; 78: 1–16.
(154) Lowe SL, Francis PT, Procter AW, Palmer AM, Davison AN, Bowen DM.
Gamma-aminobutyric acid concentration in brain tissue at two stages of
Alzheimer's disease. *Brain* 1988; 111: 785–99.
(155) Tamminga CA, Foster NL, Fedio P, Bird ED, Chase TN. Alzheimer's disease:
Low cerebral somatostatin levels correlate with impaired cognitive function and
cortical metabolism. *Neurology* 1987; 37: 161–5.

92

(156) Dawbarn D, Rossor MN, Mountjoy CQ, Roth M, Emson PC. Decreased somatostatin immunoreactivity but not neuropeptide Y immunoreactivity in cerebral cortex in senile dementia of Alzheimer type. *Neurosci Lett* 1986; 70: 154–9.
(157) Foster NL, Tamminga CA, O'Donahue TL, Tanimoto K, Bird ED, Chase TN. Brain choline acetyltransferase activity and neuropeptide Y concentrations in Alzheimer's disease. *Neurosci Lett* 1986; 63: 71–5.
(158) Nakamura S, Vincent SR. Somatostatin and neuropeptide Y immunoreactive neurones in the neocortex in senile dementia of Alzheimer type. *Brain Res* 1986; 370: 11–20.
(159) Rossor MN, Fahrenkrug J, Emson P, Mountjoy C, Iversen L, Roth M. Reduced cortical choline acetyltransferase activity in senile dementia of Alzheimer type is not accompanied by changes in vasoactive intestinal polypeptide. *Brain Res* 1980; 201: 249–53.
(160) Perry RH, Dockray GJ, Dimaline R, Perry EK, Blessed G, Tomlinson BE. Neuropeptides in Alzheimer's disease, depression and schizophrenia. A post mortem analysis of vasoactive intestinal polypeptide and cholecystokinin in cerebral cortex. *J Neurol Sci* 1981; 51: 465–72.
(161) Ferrier IN, Cross AJ, Johnson HA et al. Neuropeptides in Alzheimer type dementia. *J Neurol Sci* 1983; 62: 159–70.
(162) Mazurek MF, Beal MF, Malloy JR, Martin JB. Vasoactive intestinal peptide immunoreactivity in Alzheimer cerebral cortex. *Ann Neurol* 1986; 20: 126.
(163) Bissette G, Reynolds GP, Kilts CD, Widerlöv E, Nemeroff CB. Corticotropin-releasing factor-like immunoreactivity in senile dementia of the Alzheimer type. *JAMA* 1985; 254: 3067–9.
(164) DeSouza EB, Whitehouse PJ, Kuhar MJ, Price DL, Vale WW. Reciprocal changes in corticotropin-releasing factor (CRF)-like immunoreactivity and CRF receptors in cerebral cortex of Alzheimer's disease. *Nature* 1986; 319: 593–5.
(165) Kelley M, Kowall N. Corticotropin-releasing factor immunoreactive neurons persist throughout the brain in Alzheimer's disease. *Brain Res* 1989; 501: 392–6.
(166) Whitehouse PJ, Vale WW, Zweig RM et al. Reductions in corticotropin releasing factor-like immunoreactivity in cerebral cortex in Alzheimer's disease, Parkinson's disease, and progressive supranuclear palsy. *Neurology* 1987; 37: 905–9.
(167) Rossor MN, Rehfeld JF, Emson PC, Mountjoy CQ, Roth M, Iversen LL. Normal cortical concentrations of cholecystokinin-like immunoreactivity with reduced choline acetyltransferase activity in senile dementia of the Alzheimer type. *Life Sci* 1981; 29: 405–10.
(168) Crystal HA, Davies P. Cortical substance P-like immunoreactivity in cases of Alzheimer's disease and senile dementia of the Alzheimer type. *J Neurochem* 1982; 38: 1781–4.
(169) Chu DCM, Penney JB, Young AB. Cortical GABA$_B$ and GABA$_A$ receptors in Alzheimer's disease: A quantitative autoradiographic study. *Neurology* 1987; 37: 1454–9.
(170) Reisine TD, Yamamura HI, Bird ED, Spokes E, Enna SJ. Pre- and postsynap-

tic neurochemical alterations in Alzheimer's disease. *Brain Res* 1978; 159: 477–81.

(171) Shimohama S, Taniguchi T, Fujiwara M, Kameyama M. Changes in benzodiazepine receptors in Alzheimer-type dementia. *Ann Neurol* 1988; 23: 404–6.

(172) Beal MF, Mazurek MT, Tran VT, Chattha GK, Bird ED, Martin JB. Somatostatin receptors are reduced in cerebral cortex in Alzheimer's disease. *Science* 1985; 229: 289–91.

(173) Epelbaum J, Enjalbert A, Hamon M, Kordon C, Lamour Y. Somatostatin binding sites are decreased in rat frontal cortex after lesion of the ascending cholinergic fibres from the nucleus basalis magnocellulairs [Abstract]. *Soc Neurosci* 1985; 11: 416.

(174) Levitzki A. Regulation of hormone-sensitive adenylate cyclase. *Trends Pharmacol Sci* 1987; 8: 299–303.

(175) Worley PF, Baraban MJ, Snyder SH. Beyond receptors: multiple second messenger systems in brain. *Ann Neurol* 1987; 21: 217–29.

(176) Poat JA, Cripps HE, Iversen LL. Differences between high-affinity forskolin binding sites in dopamine-rich and other regions of rat brain. *Proc Natl Acad Sci USA* 1988; 85: 3216–20.

(177) Dewar D, Horsburgh K. Graham DI, Brooks DN, McCulloch J. Selective alterations of high affinity [^{3}H]-forskolin binding sites in Alzheimer's Disease: A quantitative autoradiographic study. *Brain Res* 1990; in press.

(178) Danielsson E, Eckernas S-A, Westlind-Danielsson A et al. VIP sensitive adenylate cyclase, guanylate cyclase, muscarinic receptors, choline acetyltransferase and acetylcholinesterase, in brain tissue afflicted by Alzheimer's disease/senile dementia of the Alzheimer type. *Neurobiol Aging* 1987; 9: 153–62.

(179) Nicoletti F, Wroblewski JT, Novelli A, Guidotti AL, Costa E. Excitatory amino acid signal transduction in cerebellar cell cultures. *Func Neurol* 1986; 1: 345–9.

(180) Fisher SK, Agranoff BW. Receptor activation and inositol lipid hydrolysis in neural tissues. *J Neurochem* 1987; 48: 999–1017.

(181) Smith CJ, Perry EK, Perry RH, Fairbairn AF, Birdsall NJM. Guanine nucleotide modulation of muscarinic cholinergic receptor binding in postmortem human brain – a preliminary study in Alzheimer's disease. *Neurosci Lett* 1987; 82: 227–32.

(182) Scarth BJ, Jhamandas K, Boegman RJ, Beninger RJ, Reynolds JN. Cortical muscarinic receptor function following quinolinic acid-induced lesion of the nucleus basalis magnocellularis. *Exp Neurol* 1989; 103: 158–64.

(183) Reed LJ, de Belleroche J. Increased polyphosphoinositide responsiveness in the cerebral cortex induced by cholinergic denervation. *J Neurochem* 1988; 50: 1566–71.

(184) Stokes CE, Hawthorne JN. Reduced phosphoinositide concentrations in anterior temporal cortex of Alzheimer-diseased brains. *J Neurochem* 1987; 48: 1018–21.

(185) Young, LT, Kish SJ, Li PP, Warsh JJ. Decreased brain [^{3}H]-inositol 1,4,5-triphosphate binding in Alzheimer's disease. *Neurosci Lett* 1988; 94: 198–202.

(186) Cole G, Dobkins KR, Hansen LA, Terry RD, Saitoh T. Decreased levels of protein kinase C in Alzheimer brain. *Brain Res* 1988; 452: 165–74.

Molecular neuropathology of Alzheimer's disease

M GOEDERT, M C POTIER AND M G SPILLANTINI

Introduction

Alzheimer's disease is characterized by a loss of memory and other cognitive functions, resulting in severe dementia and, ultimately, death[1]. It is a common disease, affecting 0.5–1% of the population in the Western world; its cause is unknown and there exists no generally effective treatment. Most cases of Alzheimer's disease appear to be sporadic and its incidence increases dramatically with age. However, there exist familial forms of the disease and the defect responsible for one such form with an onset around the age of 40 has been linked to the centromeric region of chromosome 21[2-4]. This finding is in line with the fact that the vast majority of patients with trisomy 21 over 35 years of age also develop the characteristic neuropathological features of Alzheimer's disease[5]. Age, the familial Alzheimer's disease locus and Down's syndrome thus constitute the three known risk factors of Alzheimer's disease.

Neuropathologically, Alzheimer's disease is characterized by abundant amyloid plaques and neurofibrillary tangles located mostly in cerebral cortex and hippocampus, as well as in some subcortical nuclei, such as amygdala, nucleus basalis of Meynert and locus coeruleus (Fig. 1). Small numbers of plaques and tangles accompany apparently normal aging in a majority of individuals, indicating that the difference with Alzheimer's disease is quantitative rather than qualitative. It is hoped that a better understanding of the molecular nature of plaques and tangles will shed light on the pathogenesis of Alzheimer's disease and will, in the long run, result in an effective treatment. Amyloid plaques are always extracellular and in their mature form, consist of a dense core of amyloid fibrils. In contrast, neurofibrillary tangles are mostly intracellular and their major constituent is the paired helical filament; they are found both in abnormal neurites within neuropil and senile plaques and in nerve cell bodies. Over the past 6 years, biochemistry and molecular biology

All correspondence to: Dr M Goedert, Medical Research Council Laboratory of Molecular Biology, Hills Road, Cambridge CB2 2QH, UK.

Cambridge Medical Reviews: Neurobiology and Psychiatry Volume 1
© Cambridge University Press

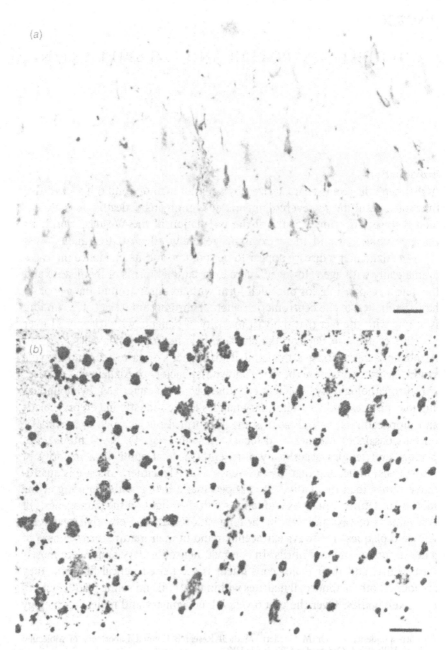

Fig. 1. Numerous neurofibrillary tangles (*a*) and amyloid plaques (*b*) in hippocampal formation from an Alzheimer's disease patient. Scale bars, 100 μm.

have permitted progress towards an understanding of the constituents of plaques and tangles and their possible mode of formation.

Beta amyloid protein and the amyloid fibril

Beta amyloid protein is the major constituent of amyloid plaques[6,7]. Protein purification led to the determination of a partial amino acid sequence, and this in turn allowed several groups to isolate cDNA clones encoding one form of the beta amyloid precursor of 695 amino acids[8-11]. Subsequently, two further forms were discovered that are produced from the same gene through alternative RNA splicing[12-14]. They are 751 or 770 amino acids in length and they differ from the first form by the presence of an extra domain encoding a serine protease inhibitor. The 751 and 770 amino acid forms differ by a stretch of 19 amino acids of unknown function. These 3 forms account for the vast majority of beta amyloid precursor mRNAs and their predicted amino acid sequences contain the entire beta amyloid sequence. A minor transcript encodes the 19 amino acids without the protease inhibitor domain, resulting in an isoform of 714 amino acids[15,16]. A fourth type of cDNA which results in a truncated beta amyloid precursor molecule without the beta amyloid sequence has also been described[17]. This isoform of 563 amino acids contains the protease inhibitor domain, but lacks 208 amino acids at the carboxy-terminus which are replaced by 20 amino acids with nucleotide homology to the Alu repeat family.

The beta amyloid precursors possess the characteristics of transmembrane proteins, with a large extracellular domain, a hydrophobic membrane-spanning region and a short cytoplasmic tail (Fig. 2)[8]. The beta amyloid protein that is deposited in large amounts in Alzheimer's disease and that forms fibrils in vitro is 42–43 amino acids long and is located towards the carboxy-terminus of the beta amyloid precursor, where its first 28 amino acids are located just outside the membrane and the remaining 14–15 amino acids in the hydrophobic transmembrane domain (Fig. 2). The major question in relation to beta amyloid deposition is thus how and why the beta amyloid precursor is cleaved out of the much larger precursor.

The molecular cloning of cDNAs encoding the beta amyloid precursor has permitted the investigation of the tissue and cellular distributions of the various mRNAs in tissues both from control patients and from patients who had died with Alzheimer's disease. Studies using probes that did not distinguish between the various beta amyloid precursor forms showed high levels of mRNA not only in the central nervous system, but also in all peripheral tissues investigated[9,10]. In situ hybridization on the brain showed that the cellular localization of beta amyloid precursor mRNAs is mostly neuronal[18,19]. This suggests that the deposition of beta amyloid in Alzheimer's disease may result from neuronal dysfunction. In cerebral cortex beta amyloid precursor mRNAs are found in pyramidal cells throughout all layers,

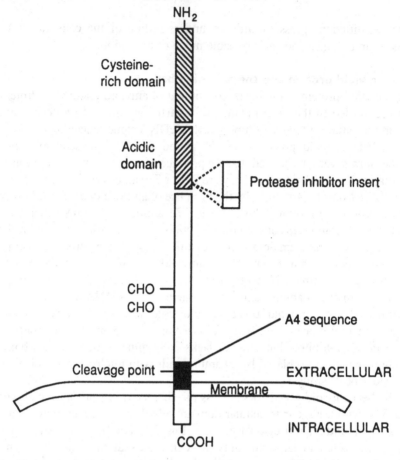

Fig. 2. Schematic drawing of the beta amyloid precursor. The amino-terminus is located outside the cell and contains a sequence with a high content of cysteine residues and a region rich in acidic residues. The protease inhibitor domain is inserted into the acidic domain. CHO, potential glycosylation sites. Constitutive processing of the precursor leads to cleavage close to the transmembrane region. The carboxy-terminus is located intracellularly. The beta amyloid sequence (A4) that gets deposited in Alzheimer's disease is marked in black.

with the largest number in layers III and V. In the hippocampal formation beta amyloid precursor mRNAs are present in granule cells in the dentate gyrus, pyramidal cells throughout all CA layers, and pyramidal cells in the subiculum (Fig. 3). The same qualitative and quantitative distribution was found in cerebral cortex and hippocampus from patients who had died with Alzheimer's disease[18,19], whereas an increase in beta amyloid precursor mRNAs in the nucleus basalis of Meynert from Alzheimer's disease patients has been reported[20]. Subsequently, it was shown that mRNAs encoding the 751- and 770-amino acid forms are found at high levels in peripheral and central tissues, whereas mRNA encoding the 695-amino acid form is found predominantly in brain[15,16,21–23]. In situ hybridization studies indicate that both types of mRNAs are expressed in the same cells in the hippocampus[23], suggesting that the presence of the protease inhibitor domain in the beta amyloid precursor is unlikely to protect the vulnerable cells from degeneration. An increasing number of studies uses RNA blotting techniques, RNase protection assays and in situ hybridization to compare the relative levels of beta amyloid precursor transcripts between brain regions from control patients and from patients who had died with Alzheimer's disease. Several studies have described a reduction in the mRNA encoding the 695 amino acid form, with no concomitant change in mRNA levels for the 751 and 770 amino acid forms[21–23]. This contrasts with studies reporting a reduction in mRNA encoding the 695 amino acid form and an increase in mRNAs for the 751 and 770 amino acid forms[15], no changes in transcript ratios[24], an increase in the 751/695 mRNA ratio when compared with controls[25], an increase in the mRNA encoding the 770 amino acid form[26] and an increase in the mRNA encoding the 563 amino acid form when compared with controls[27].

The above studies indicate that there exists a correlation between the tissue and cellular distributions of beta amyloid precursor mRNAs and the pathology of Alzheimer's disease only insofar as the cells affected by the disease produce the corresponding mRNAs. However, the distribution of the latter is much more widespread. At present, it appears unlikely that it is an overproduction of beta amyloid precursor mRNAs that leads to beta amyloid deposition in Alzheimer's disease.

Whereas the physiological role of the beta amyloid precursor in the brain is not known, significant progress has been made regarding its normal turnover and processing. After the elucidation of the nucleotide and deduced amino acid sequences of the isoforms with the protease inhibitor domain, it became apparent that these isoforms were identical with a protein previously identified through its protease inhibitory activity and called protease nexin II[28,29]. The latter is probably released into the extracellular space, where it inactivates serine proteases; this is followed by its binding to the cell as a protease/inhibitor complex, resulting in the internalization of the complex. In platelets, protease nexin II functions as an inhibitor of coagulation factor XIa, implying a role in hemostasis[30,31]. These and other[32–34] results strongly indicated the existence of soluble forms that are released from beta amyloid precursors and initial experiments suggested that this physiological cleavage might occur within the beta amyloid sequence close to the transmembrane region[34]. This has now been demonstrated directly by protein sequencing of released and membrane-bound forms following transfection of cDNA clones into embryonic kidney cells[35]. The cleavage occurs either between Gln15–Lys16 or Lys16–Leu17 of the beta amyloid sequence, implying the existence of a protease (named APP secretase) that effects this cleavage. The important implications of these results are that the normal constitutive pro-

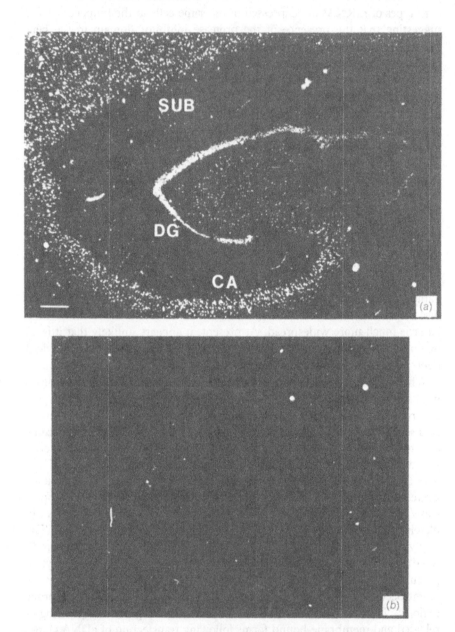

Fig. 3. Cellular localization of beta amyloid precursor mRNAs encoding the protease inhibitor domain in the hippocampal formation from a control patient.

(a), (b) Dark-field photomicrographs of hippocampal formation after hybridization with a probe in the anti-mRNA sense (a) or mRNA sense (b) orientation. (c), (d) Light-field photomicrographs of pyramidal cells in the CA3 region of the hippo-

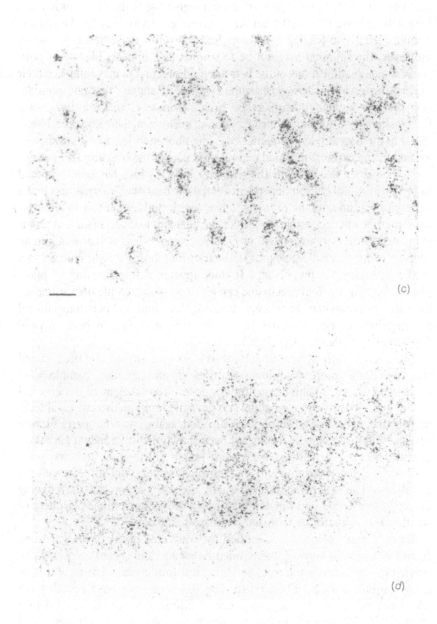

campus: (c) and granule cells in the dentate gyrus: (d) following hybridization with a probe in the anti-mRNA sense orientation. SUB, subiculum; DG, dentate gyrus; CA, cornu ammonis. Scale bars in (a) (for (a) and (b)) = 350 μm; in (c) (for (c) and (d)) = 21 μm.

cessing of the beta amyloid precursor cannot give rise to the 42–43 amino acid beta amyloid and that inefficient APP secretase activity may be the starting point for the events leading to beta amyloid deposition in Alzheimer's disease. However, the situation may not be so simple, as it appears likely that post-translational modifications of the beta amyloid precursors may influence their normal processing. There exists some evidence to suggest that phosphorylation of beta amyloid precursors by protein kinase C and multifunctional Ca^{2+}/calmodulin-dependent protein kinase results in their cleavage N-terminal to the beta amyloid sequence[36,37]. The phosphorylated residues may be located in the carboxy-terminal cytoplasmic part of the beta amyloid precursor[36]. The latter also contains the sequence NPTY which has been proposed to be involved in ligand-independent coated pit-mediated internalization of a variety of transmembrane proteins[38]. It is worth noting that this sequence is conserved in a molecule that resembles the beta amyloid precursor and that is expressed in the nervous system of *D melanogaster*[39,40], as well as in a human sperm protein that is homologous to the transmembrane/cytoplasmic domain of the beta amyloid precursor[41]. It thus appears that processing of phosphorylated beta amyloid precursors can give rise to a molecule that comprises the entire beta amyloid sequence, suggesting that abnormal post-translational modifications of beta amyloid precursors may give rise to beta amyloid deposition in Alzheimer's disease.

Over the past three years, important new information has also been gained concerning the more traditional features of the amyloid pathology of Alzheimer's disease. This is mainly due to the replacement of the classical staining methods by more sensitive and versatile immunohistochemical techniques that make use of antibodies directed against various parts of beta amyloid and its precursor. It thus has been shown that the amyloid pathology is both more severe and extensive than previously thought and that some antibodies detect predominantly a neuronal rather than an extracellular pathology. The latter result is especially relevant in view of the ongoing debate as to whether beta amyloid may reach the brain from the periphery or whether it results from a localized neuronal pathology.

Classical senile plaques as identified by Congo red or thioflavin S staining consist of a core of amyloid surrounded by an amyloid corona, as well as by tangle-bearing neurites and reactive astrocytes. Immunohistochemical studies using antibodies raised against beta amyloid sequences have revealed the additional existence of a large number of diffuse plaques (also called pre-amyloid)[42,43]. These are found in the same brain regions as senile plaques and are usually not surrounded by abnormal neurites. Moreover, diffuse plaques can also be found in brain regions devoid of classical plaques, such as basal ganglia and cerebellum[44,45]. Diffuse plaques are generally thought to represent an early stage of extracellular beta amyloid pathology. This is supported by the presence of only few amyloid fibrils in these deposits[46], indicating that diffuse plaques contain mostly beta amyloid and beta amyloid precursor epitopes that are not yet organized in fibrils. The same may be true of the senile plaque corona that reacts with beta amyloid precursor antibodies outside the beta amyloid region[47]. The existence of distinct configurational states of beta amyloid is evident from the fact that it is possible to obtain antisera directed against different parts of the beta amyloid sequence that react predominantly with different kinds of amyloid distributions in Alzheimer's disease hippocampus – namely, amyloid plaques without cores, amyloid plaques with cores, or neurofibrillary tangle-bearing bodies and cells (Fig. 4)[48]. These findings, together with the knowledge that has been gained on the processing of beta amyloid precursors, have led to the proposal of a molecular explanation of the events leading to beta amyloid deposition in Alzheimer's disease (Fig. 5)[48]. As illustrated in Figure 5(a), in the central nervous system intact beta amyloid precursors are non-amyloidogenic neuronal transmembrane proteins. In tangle-bearing cells these precursors have been cleaved to expose the amino-terminal sequence of beta amyloid itself but are not yet completely processed to beta amyloid and, moreover, are still anchored in, and distributed over the cell surface (Fig. 5(b)). Further proteolysis of the precursors would cut at the point corresponding to the carboxy-terminus of beta amyloid, freeing beta amyloid protein and leading to its deposition and aggregation in the extracellular space (Fig. 5(c) and (d)). Amyloid deposition would thus be at least a three-step process consisting of the production of an amyloidogenic protein, which is at first still located at the cell surface, and which after further proteolytic processing is released as beta amyloid that aggregates to form amyloid fibrils.

The above interpretation implies that the events leading to beta amyloid deposition in sporadic Alzheimer's disease are post-translational and that beta amyloid precursors merely constitute the substrates for pathological and so far unknown mechanisms that result in the formation of large quantities of beta amyloid. This contrasts with the case of hereditary cerebral hemorrhage with amyloidosis of the Dutch type, a rare inherited disease that is characterized by extensive beta amyloid deposition in small leptomeningeal arteries and cortical arterioles, leading to death through cerebral hemorrhage[49,50]. Some of these patients also develop diffuse beta amyloid deposits in the cerebral cortex, although dementia and neurofibrillary tangles are not observed. Genetic linkage analysis in two of the Dutch families has shown that the beta amyloid precursor gene is closely linked to the disease locus[51], suggesting that a mutation in this gene may cause the disease. This has now been demonstrated in that DNA sequencing detected a point mutation in the beta amyloid precursor coding region that causes the substitution of a glutamine for a glutamic residue at position 22 of beta amyloid[52]. It is interesting to note that the mutation is located only 6 amino acids downstream of the constitutive processing cleavage site.

M Goedert, M C Potier & M G Spillantini

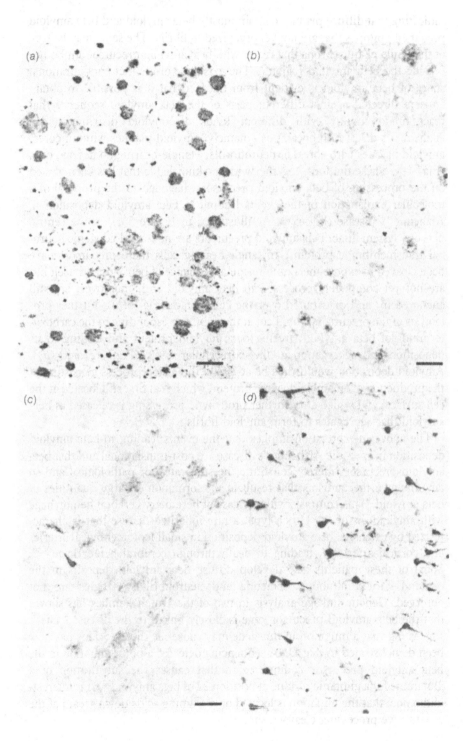

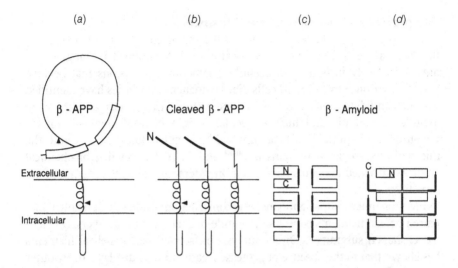

Fig. 5. Diagram of proposed stages leading to the deposition of beta amyloid in the hippocampal formation of Alzheimer's disease patients, based on the staining pattern observed with different anti-beta amyloid antibodies (see Fig. 4). (a) Schematic drawing (not to scale) of the intact beta amyloid precursor protein as a non-amyloidogenic transmembrane protein. (b) The first proteolytic cleavage produces the amino-terminus of beta amyloid, leading to the formation of an amyloidogenic protein that is immunoreactive with an antibody directed against amino acids 1–12 of beta amyloid, but is still membrane-bound and dispersed. (c) The second proteolytic cleavage frees the carboxy-terminus of beta amyloid, leading to the formation and aggregation of beta amyloid that is immunoreactive with an antibody directed against amino acids 17–24 of beta amyloid. (d) More highly condensed aggregates of beta amyloid that are immunoreactive with an antibody directed against amino acids 28–40 of beta amyloid. The drawings in (c) and (d) are highly schematic and are only meant to illustrate different epitope availabilities in condensing and condensed beta amyloid. The detailed configuration(s) of beta amyloid is not known. Positions of positive epitopes are marked by thickened lines.

Fig. 4. Labelling of subiculum/entorhinal cortex from Alzheimer's disease patients with antibodies raised against different parts of the beta amyloid sequence. (a) An antibody directed against amino acids 17–24 stains amyloid plaques and diffuse amyloid deposits. (b) An antibody directed against amino acids 28–40 stains plaque cores strongly and the rest of the plaques more weakly, but not diffuse amyloid deposits. (c) An antibody directed against amino acids 1–12 stains diffuse amyloid deposits weakly and a pyramid cell (arrowhead). (d) The same antibody as in (c) stains numerous nerve cells throughout the entorhinal cortex. These are tangle-bearing cells, as demonstrated by tau staining of serial sections from this area (data not shown). Bars = 80 μm.

Tau protein and the paired helical filament
The paired helical filament constitutes the major component of the neuro-fibrillary tangle of Alzheimer's disease (Fig. 6)[53]. Neurofibrillary tangles start out as relatively insoluble intracellular filamentous inclusions that become extracellular once the affected cells die. Histochemical studies have identified various candidate molecules as components of neurofibrillary tangles; these include the middle and high molecular weight neurofilament subunits[54], vimentin[55], ubiquitin[56,57], beta amyloid[58], acetylcholinesterase[59], and the microtubule-associated proteins tau[60-64] and MAP2[65]. Detailed biochemical studies of isolated filaments have so far only demonstrated the presence of tau protein.

Electron microscopic and image reconstruction studies have shown that paired helical filaments consist of a double-helical stack of transversely orien-ted C-shaped subunits[66]. Direct analysis of isolated paired helical filaments has shown that in the absence of protease treatment they display a fuzzy outer coat which is removed by pronase to leave a protease-resistant core that retains the characteristic paired helical filament morphology[67]. A monoclonal antibody raised against purified paired helical filament core preparations was found to identify core filaments clearly and to label protein fragments isolated from paired helical filament core preparations[68]. This established a link between the paired helical filament core as a morphological entity and specific peptides extracted from it. Two different amino acid sequences were obtained from a 9.5 kd band and these led to the cloning and sequencing of cDNAs, which were shown to encode an isoform of the microtubule-associated protein tau of 352 amino acids[69]. Subsequently, an isoform of 383 amino acids was identified[70,71]. The most striking feature of the tau protein sequence is the presence of tandem repeats of 31 or 32 amino acids located in the carboxy-terminal half and containing a characteristic Pro–Gly–Gly–Gly motif; the repeats which are rich in basic amino acids are involved in the binding of tau to an acidic domain of tubulin and in promoting the in vitro assembly of tubulin into microtubules[72,73]. The smaller protein contains three and the larger 4 of these repeats that are produced from a single gene through alterna-tive RNA splicing[70]. The extra repeat in the 4-repeat isoform is inserted within the first repeat of the 3-repeat isoform in a way that preserves the periodic pattern. Twelve residues are completely conserved between the 4 repeats and a further 4 residues show conservative changes. Similar microtubule-binding repeats are found in the carboxy-terminal region of the high-molecular weight microtubule-associated proteins MAP2[74] and MAP-U[75]. MAP2 is also nervous system-specific, whereas MAP-U shows a ubiquitous distribution.

The existence of additional tau protein isoforms with insertions of 29 or 58 amino acids in the amino-terminal half has been inferred from molecular cloning studies[76]; they exist in combination with 3 and 4 repeat-containing

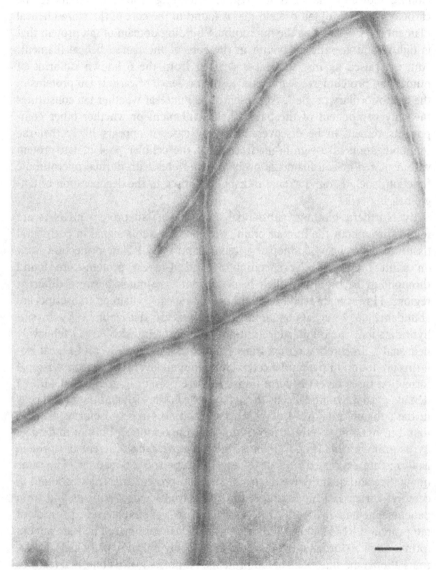

Fig. 6. Isolated paired helical filaments shown by electron microscopy after negative staining. Scale bar, 100 nm.

isoforms, implying the existence of at least 6 isoforms of human tau protein. Similar sequences have also been described in mouse[77], rat[78] and cow[79,80]. The comparison of the protein sequences obtained from the paired helical filament core with that of the sequence of tau protein as deduced by cDNA cloning indicates that it is the region extending from the repeats to the carboxy-terminus of tau protein that is found in the core of the paired helical filament[68-70,81]. It is thus the microtubule-binding domain of tau protein that is tightly and specifically bound in the core of the paired helical filament. Antisera raised against sequences derived from the 6 known isoforms of human tau protein have demonstrated the presence of various tau proteins in the neurofibrillary tangle[76]. At present, it is not clear whether tau constitutes the only component of the paired helical filament or whether other components remain to be discovered. In any case, it appears likely that the immobilization of a significant fraction of the cellular pool of tau protein within paired helical filaments probably interferes with normal microtubule function, such as rapid axonal transport, leading to the degeneration of tangle-bearing cells.

By Northern blotting, substantial amounts of tau protein mRNAs are found throughout the human brain, with no detectable signal in peripheral tissues, such as heart, kidney or adrenal gland[69]. By RNase protection assay on adult brain mRNAs encoding 3- and 4-repeat proteins are found throughout the brain and their levels do not vary much between different regions. However, in fetal brain, although 3 repeat-containing transcripts are abundant, no 4 repeat-containing transcripts are detectable[70]. By in situ hybridization, the cellular localization of tau protein mRNAs is exclusively neuronal[70]. In cerebral cortex transcripts encoding either 3- or 4-repeat isoforms are found in pyramidal cells throughout all layers. In the hippocampal formation three repeat isoform transcripts are present in granule cells in the dentate gyrus, pyramidal cells throughout the CA layers, and pyramidal cells in the subiculum (Fig. 7). Transcripts encoding 4-repeat isoforms are also found in pyramidal cells in subiculum and hippocampus, but not in dentate gyrus granule cells (Fig. 7). Thus, mRNAs encoding different tau protein isoforms are expressed in a stage- and cell type-specific manner. The same qualitative and quantitative distribution of tau protein mRNAs was found in cerebral cortex and hippocampal formation from control patients and from patients who had died with Alzheimer's disease[76]. A simple overexpression of tau protein mRNAs is thus unlikely to be the cause of paired helical filament formation. The formation of the latter is probably linked to pathological post-translational modifications of tau proteins. At present, two abnormal features of tau proteins in Alzheimer's disease are known which might be directly related to the formation of paired helical filaments. These are an abnormal distribution within nerve cells and abnormal states of phosphorylation.

Tau proteins and MAP2 are major microtubule-associated proteins of the nervous system. When visualized in normal nerve cells by immuno-histochemical techniques they display a striking complementary distribution, with tau proteins being found in axons and MAP2 in dendrites[82,83]. MAP2 is composed of at least three isoforms that appear to be generated from a single gene through alternative RNA splicing[74,84]. In the rat, MAP2b is a protein of 280 kd apparent molecular weight that is expressed throughout brain development. MAP2a is slightly larger than MAP2b; it appears in cerebral cortex around post-natal day 12 and is found in adult nerve cells. A 70 kd MAP2 variant, called MAP2c, is expressed during embryonic brain development and until postnatal day 10. The MAP2 cDNA clones that have been isolated encode MAP2b or MAP2c[85]; at present, the difference between MAP2a and MAP2b is not known. By in situ hybridization on brain sections, MAP2 mRNA is not only found in neuronal cell bodies, but also in dendrites[86], indicating that the dendritic localization of MAP2 is paralleled by the association of MAP2 mRNA with the dendritic cytoplasm. This suggests that MAP2 may owe its restricted distribution to the sequestration of its mRNA within the dendrite.

There also exists evidence to indicate that the information for MAP2 segregation may reside within the protein itself. Biotinylated MAP2, when microinjected into nerve cells maintained in primary culture, becomes uniformly distributed to axons and dendrites[87]. However, within 1 day after injection, the MAP2 disappears from the axons, indicating the correct segregation. Similarly, when biotinylated tau is microinjected, it also is uniformly distributed initially, only to become segregated to the axon at a later stage[88]. The mechanisms underlying the segregation of MAP2 and tau are unknown; the above results suggest a greater lability of each protein in the cellular compartment it is normally not found in. An understanding of the mechanisms underlying the polarity of tau and MAP2 may be directly relevant to the pathogenesis of Alzheimer's disease, since tau is found in an insoluble form within the somatodendritic compartment of tangle-bearing nerve cells (Fig. 7). The question therefore arises why a substantial proportion of the otherwise soluble axonal tau protein becomes immobilized in an insoluble form within the somatodendritic compartment of certain nerve cells.

In normal brain, tau protein exists as several molecular species, as evidenced by the fact that it runs as 4–5 discrete bands on denaturing gels. Human tau isoforms expressed in *E. coli* give a characteristic set of six bands (Fig. 8)[89]. A comparison of the pattern of recombinant tau isoforms with that of native tau has shown that the 4 major tau isoforms in adult human brain correspond to isoforms with three repeats and no inserts, 4 repeats and no amino-terminal insertions, 3 repeats and the short amino-terminal insertion and 4 repeats and the short amino-terminal insertion. Phosphorylation also contributes to the complex pattern of tau bands, as some bands exhibit an increased mobility on denaturing gels following alkaline phosphatase treatment[30]. Recombinant tau proteins can be phosphorylated in vitro by cAMP-dependent protein kinase, Ca^{2+}/calmodulin-dependent protein kinase,

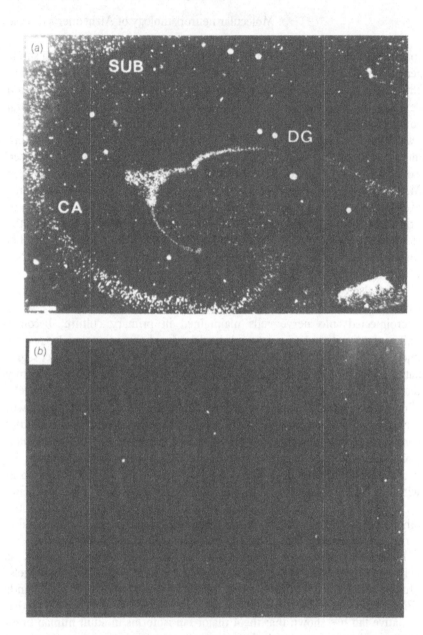

Fig. 7. Cellular localization of tau protein transcripts encoding isoforms with three or four repeats in the hippocampal formation from a control patient. (*a*), (*b*) Dark-field photomicrographs of hippocampal formation after hybridization with an oligonucleotide probe specific for transcripts encoding three repeat-containing isoforms labelled in the anti-mRNA sense orientation (*a*) or mRNA sense (*b*) orientation. (*c*), (*d*) Dentate gyrus sections hybridized with probes specific for transcripts encoding three repeat (*c*) or four repeat (*d*)- containing isoforms. Granule cells are labelled in (*c*),

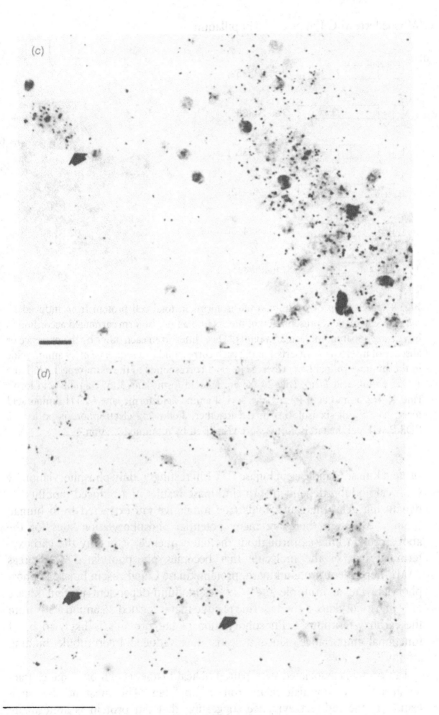

but not in (*d*). SUB, subiculum; DG, dentate gyrus; CA, cornu ammonis. Scale bars
in (*a*) (for (*a*) and (*b*)) = 350 μm; in (*c*) for (*c*) and (*d*) = 25 μm.

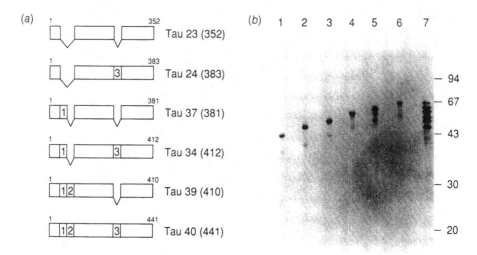

Fig. 8. Expression of six human tau isoforms in total cell protein from induced *E. coli*. (*a*) Schematic representation of the six human tau isoforms arranged according to increasing apparent molecular weights. They differ from each other by the presence or absence of inserts 1–3. Inserts 1 and 2 each correspond to a sequence of 29 amino acids in the amino-terminal half, whereas insert 3 corresponds to the extra repeat. (*b*) Lane 1, 352 amino acid form; lane 2, 383 amino acid form; lane 3, 381 amino acid form; lane 4, 412 amino acid form; lane 5, 410 amino acid form; lane 6, 441 amino acid form; lane 7, all six isoforms mixed together. Following electrophoresis on a 10% SDS/PAGE gel the tau isoforms were visualized by immunodetection.

protein kinase C and casein kinase II[30]. Interestingly, only phosphorylation by Ca^{2+}/calmodulin-dependent protein kinase results in a reduced mobility on denaturing gels; the same holds true for native tau extracted from human brain[91]. Although there are many potential phosphorylation sites for the above protein kinases throughout the tau sequence, it is only the carboxy-terminal half of the molecule that becomes phosphorylated[90]. Whereas cAMP-dependent protein kinase, protein kinase C and casein kinase II phosphorylate tau at multiple sites Ca^{2+}/calmodulin-dependent protein kinase only phosphorylates a single serine residue that is located 26 amino acids from the carboxy-terminus[90]. Phosphorylation of tau proteins is likely to be of functional importance, since it leads to a reduced microtubule binding affinity[92].

Tau proteins associated with paired helical filaments exhibit some characteristics that distinguish them from normal tau. The most notable such feature is the indirect evidence suggesting that tau protein is abnormally phosphorylated in Alzheimer's disease. Histologically, it has been shown that certain tau antibodies only label neurofibrillary tangles following the pretreat-

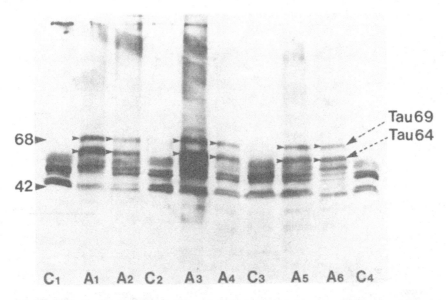

Fig. 9. Visualization by immunodetection of tau proteins in temporal cortex extracts from control (C1–C4) and Alzheimer's disease (A1–A6) patients. Note that Tau 64 and 69 are only present in Alzheimer brain homogenates.

ment of tissue sections with alkaline phosphatase[93]. Biochemically, it has been reported that in Alzheimer's disease the extraction of sodium dodecylsulphate-soluble tau protein from affected brain regions exhibits the presence of two bands of 64 and 69 kd that are not observed in non-affected brain regions or in brain regions from control patients (Fig. 9)[94,95]. These molecular species are abnormally phosphorylated, as they show an increased gel mobility following alkaline phosphatase treatment. It is interesting to note that these abnormal tau forms are soluble in sodium dodecylsulphate, unlike a large proportion of paired helical filaments[96]. It is therefore conceivable that they represent abnormal tau species prior to their incorporation into paired helical filaments; alternatively, they may be derived from the population of paired helical filaments that is soluble in sodium dodecylsulphate[97]. Since paired helical filaments are found both intra- and extracellularly it is possible that the cytoplasmic population is soluble in sodium dodecylsulphate, whereas the extracellular population which may be more extensively cross-linked is insoluble. Only two abnormal tau species are consistently observed, implying that at least two tau isoforms are abnormally phosphorylated in a way such as to result in a reduced gel mobility. The latter is characteristic of the phosphorylation of a single serine residue in tau by Ca^{2+}/calmodulin-dependent

M Goedert, MC Potier & MG Spillantini

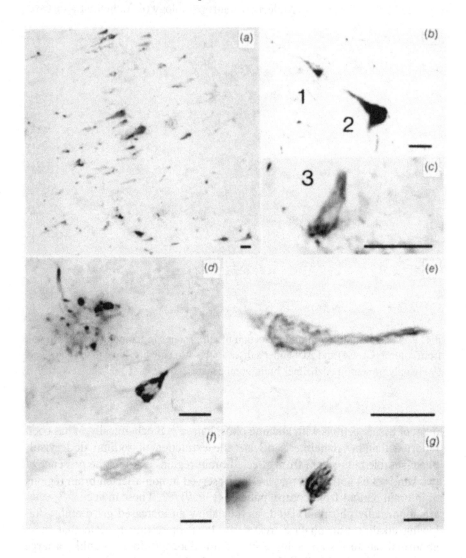

Fig. 10. Double-labelling of subiculum/entorhinal cortex from Alzheimer's disease patients with an antibody directed against amino acids 1–12 of beta amyloid and a tau protein antibody. *(a) Beta amyloid antibody (brown) followed by tau antibody (blue)* Numerous tau-positive pyramidal cells are of normal size and shape and are therefore presumably intact tangle-bearing cells. On the other hand, while many of the beta amyloid-positive cells are of normal size and shape, a significant number are much enlarged, suggesting that the original cell may already be disrupted. In general, the whole cell stains either brown or blue, giving the impression of two non-overlapping populations, but there are a number that are partially covered by both antibodies (see *(b)* and *(c)*). Nerve cells double-labelled in their entirety are only observed when the tau antibody is used first and the beta amyloid antibody is used second (see *(d)* and

114

protein kinase, suggesting a role for a protein kinase that phosphorylates this site in the generation of the abnormal tau forms observed in affected brain regions in Alzheimer's disease.

Histological studies have indicated that the beta amyloid and tau pathologies, although biochemically distinct, may be closely related in origin (Fig. 10)[98]. Double-labelling of hippocampal sections from Alzheimer's disease patients using antibodies raised against the amino-terminus of beta amyloid and against tau protein sequences has demonstrated the presence of tangle-bearing objects that were either single-labelled by tau antibodies or double-labelled by both antibodies[98]. The single-labelled tangle-bearing objects were invariably small and appeared to be intact pyramidal cells, whereas double-labelled tangle-bearing objects were of all sizes, consistent with their predominant extracellular nature. However, some nerve cells were double-labelled with both antibodies, indicating that apparently intact, but tangle-bearing, cells can also be associated with beta amyloid staining. In addition to fully double-labelled cells, a number of tau-positive cells were found that were only partially stained by the beta amyloid antibody. These cells probably represent intermediates between cells positive only for tau and fully double-labelled cells (Fig. 10). Importantly, in all cases studied, the region of staining of beta amyloid sequences was outside that of tau staining. Moreover, the order of the antibodies was important, in that fully double-labelled objects were only observed when tau antibodies were used first. The inability of tau antibodies to penetrate when the beta amyloid antibody was used first was presumably due to the 3,3-diaminobenzidine precipitate covering the outside of the cell and thus this also indicates that the beta amyloid sequences are peripheral to tau.

(e)). (b) and (c) Beta amyloid antibody (brown) followed by tau antibody (blue) A number of tangle-bearing cells are stained with both antibodies when the beta amyloid-positive material does not cover the whole cell. 1, Part of the cell body is beta amyloid-positive, whereas the region of the apical dendrite is only tau-positive; 2, beta amyloid-positive nerve cell of the enlarged type, as shown in (a); 3, tangle-bearing tau-positive cell partially covered with beta amyloid-positive material. (d) and (e) Tau antibody (brown) followed by beta amyloid antibody (blue) Inversion of the order of antibodies with respect to (a)–(c) leads to double-labelling of some apparently intact tangle-bearing pyramidal cells. The beta amyloid-positive amyloid material is on the outside of the tau-positive material, as can be confirmed by focusing through the thickness of the 40 μm section. (f) and (g) Tau antibody (brown) followed by beta amyloid antibody (blue) Extracellular tangles are stained by both antibodies when the order of the antibodies is the same as in (d) and (e), and the beta amyloid staining is invariably peripheral to the tau staining. Inversion in the order of antibodies gives only beta amyloid staining, consistent with its peripheral location blocking access to the interior. Scale bar = 35 μm.

M Goedert, M C Potier & M G Spillantini

It thus appears likely that the events leading to plaque and tangle formation might be related. One might envisage a connection through a biochemical link between the cytoplasmic tails of beta amyloid precursors and components of the cytoskeleton, which, if disturbed, leads to abnormal changes in both systems.

Conclusion

Over the past few years, research into the etiology and pathogenesis of Alzheimer's disease has progressed from a necessary but limited descriptive stage to a more mechanistic phase. This has already provided important insights into the nature of the components of plaques and tangles and has opened the way to an understanding of their mode of formation. Future research will have to discover the nature of these factors. This approach, which starts at the end-stages of the disease process, is being complemented by a different approach which makes use of the existence of familial forms of Alzheimer's disease. The aim there is to identify the genes that cause the disease in these families. It can be confidently expected that the convergence of these two approaches will lead to a true understanding of the etiology and pathogenesis of Alzheimer's disease in the not too distant future.

Acknowledgements

We thank Dr RA Crowther for providing Figure 6 and Dr A Delacourte for providing Figure 9.

References

(1) Alzheimer A. Über eine eigenartige Erkrankung der Hirnrinde. *Alleg Z Psychiat* 1907; 64: 146–8.
(2) St George-Hyslop PH, Tanzi RE, Polinsky RJ, Haines JL, Nee L, Watkins PC et al. The genetic defect causing familial Alzheimer's disease maps to chromosome 21. *Science* 1987; 235: 885–90.
(3) Goate AM, Owen JM, James LA, Mullan MJ, Rossor MN, Haynes AR et al. Predisposing locus for Alzheimer's disease on chromosome 21. *Lancet* 1989; i: 352–5.
(4) St George-Hyslop PH, Haines JL, Farrer LA, Polinsky R, Van Broeckhoven C, Goate A et al. Genetic linkage studies suggest that Alzheimer's disease is not a homogeneous disorder. *Nature* 1990; 347: 194–7.
(5) Jervis GA. Early senile dementia in mongoloid idiocy. *Am J Psychiat* 1948; 105: 102–6.
(6) Glenner GG, Wong CW. Alzheimer's disease: Initial report of the purification and characterization of a novel cerebrovascular amyloid protein. *Biochem Biophys Res Commun* 1984; 112: 885–90.
(7) Masters CL, Simms G, Weinman NA, Multhaup G, McDonald BL, Beyreuther K. Amyloid plaque core protein in Alzheimer's disease and Down syndrome. *Proc Natl Acad Sci USA* 1985; 82: 4245–9.

(8) Kang J, Lemaire HG, Unterbeck A, Salbaum JM, Masters CL, Grzeschik KH et al. The precursor of Alzheimer's disease amyloid A4 resembles a cell-surface receptor. *Nature* 1987; 325: 733–6.

(9) Tanzi RE, Gusella JF, Watkins PC, Bruns GAP, St George-Hyslop PH, Van Keuren ML et al. Amyloid beta protein gene: cDNA, mRNA distribution and genetic linkage near the Alzheimer locus. *Science* 1987; 235: 880–4.

(10) Goldgaber D, Lerman MI, McBride OW, Saffiotti U, Gajdusek DC. Characterization and chromosomal localization of a cDNA encoding brain amyloid of Alzheimer's disease. *Science* 1987; 235: 877–80.

(11) Robakis N, Ramakrishna N, Wolfe G, Wisniewski HN. Molecular cloning and characterization of a cDNA encoding the cerebrovascular and the neuritic plaque amyloid peptides. *Proc Natl Acad Sci USA* 1987; 84: 4190–4.

(12) Ponte P, Gonzalez-De Whitt P, Schilling J, Miller J, Hsu D, Greenberg D et al. A new A4 amyloid mRNA contains a domain homologous to serine protease inhibitors. *Nature* 1988; 331: 525–7.

(13) Tanzi RE, McClatchey AI, Lamperti ED, Villa-Komaroff L, Gusella JF, Neve RL. Protease inhibitor domain encoded by an amyloid protein precursor mRNA associated with Alzheimer's disease. *Nature* 1988; 331: 528–30.

(14) Kitaguchi N, Takahashi Y, Tokushima Y, Shiojiri S, Ito H. Novel precursor of Alzheimer's disease amyloid protein shows protease inhibitor activity. *Nature* 1988; 331: 530–2.

(15) Kang J, Müller-Hill B. Differential splicing of Alzheimer's disease amyloid A4 precursor RNA in rat tissues: preA4695 mRNA is predominantly produced in rat and human brain. *Biochem Biophys Res Commun* 1990; 166: 1192–200.

(16) Golde TE, Estus S, Usiak M, Younkin LH, Younkin SG. Expression of beta amyloid protein precursor mRNAs: recognition of a novel alternatively spliced form and quantitation in Alzheimer's disease using PCR. *Neuron* 1990; 4: 253–67.

(17) De Sauvage F, Octave JN. A novel mRNA of the A4 amyloid precursor gene coding for a possibly secreted protein. *Science* 1989; 245: 651–3.

(18) Bahmanyar S, Higgins GA, Goldgaber D, Lewis DA, Morrison JH, Wilson MC et al. Localization of amyloid beta protein mRNA in brains from patients with Alzheimer's disease. *Science* 1987; 237: 77–80.

(19) Goedert M. Neuronal distribution of amyloid beta protein precursor mRNA in normal human brain and in Alzheimer's disease. *EMBO J* 1987; 68: 3627–32.

(20) Cohen ML, Golde TE, Usiak MF, Younkin LH, Younkin SG. *In situ* hybridization of nucleus basalis neurons shows increased beta amyloid mRNA in Alzheimer's disease. *Proc Natl Acad Sci USA* 1988; 85: 1227–31.

(21) Neve RL, Finch EA, Dawes LR. Expression of the Alzheimer amyloid precursor gene transcripts in the human brain. *Neuron* 1988; 1: 669–77.

(22) Johnson SA, Rogers J, Finch CE. APP695 transcript prevalence is selectively reduced during Alzheimer's disease in cortex and hippocampus but not in cerebellum. *Neurobiol Aging* 1989; 10: 267–72.

(23) Spillantini MG, Hunt SP, Ulrich J, Goedert M. Expression and cellular localization of amyloid beta protein precursor transcripts in normal human brain and in Alzheimer's disease. *Mol Brain Res* 1989; 6: 143–50.

(24) Koo EH, Sisodia SS, Cork LC, Unterbeck A, Bayney RM, Price DL. Differential expression of amyloid precursor protein mRNAs in cases of Alzheimer's disease and in aged nonhuman primates. *Neuron* 1990; 2: 97–104.

(25) Johnson SA, McNeill T, Cordell B, Finch CE. Relation of neuronal APP-751/APP-695 mRNA ratio and neuritic plaque density in Alzheimer's disease. *Science* 1990; 248: 854–7.

(26) Tanaka S, Nakamura S, Ueda K, Kameyama M, Shiojiri S, Takahashi Y et al. Three types of amyloid protein precursor mRNA in human brain: their differential expression in Alzheimer's disease. *Biochem Biophys Res Commun* 1988; 157: 472–9.

(27) Neve RL, Rogers J, Higgins GA. The Alzheimer amyloid precursor-related transcript lacking the beta/A4 sequence is specifically increased in Alzheimer's disease brain. *Neuron* 1990; 5: 329–38.

(28) Oltersdorf T, Fritz LC, Schenk DB, Lieberburg I, Johnson-Wood KL, Beattie EC et al. The secreted form of the Alzheimer's disease amyloid precursor protein with the Kunitz domain is protease nexin II. *Nature* 1989; 341: 144–7.

(29) Van Nostrand WE, Wagner SL, Suzuki M, Choi BH, Farrow JS, Geddes JW et al. Protease nexin II, a potent antichymotrypsin shows identity to amyloid beta protein precursor. *Nature* 1989; 341: 546–8.

(30) Van Nostrand WE, Schmaier AH, Farrow JS, Cunningham DD. Protease nexin II (Amyloid beta protein precursor): A platelet alpha-granule protein. *Science* 1990; 248: 745–8.

(31) Smith RP, Higuchi DA, Broze GJ. Platelet coagulation factor XIa-inhibitor, a form of Alzheimer amyloid precursor protein. *Science* 1990; 248: 1126–8.

(32) Weidemann A, König G, Bunke D, Fisher P, Salbaum M, Masters CL et al. Identification, biogenesis and localization of precursors of Alzheimer's disease A4 amyloid protein. *Cell* 1989; 57: 115–26.

(33) Palmert MR, Podlisny MB, Witker DS, Oltersdorf T, Younkin LH, Selkoe DJ et al. The beta amyloid protein precursor of Alzheimer disease has soluble derivatives found in human brain and cerebrospinal fluid. *Proc Natl Acad Sci USA* 1989; 86: 6338–42.

(34) Sisodia SS, Koo EH, Beyreuther K, Unterbeck A, Price DL. Evidence that beta amyloid protein in Alzheimer's disease is not derived by normal processing. *Science* 1990; 248: 492–5.

(35) Esch FS, Keim PS, Beattie EC, Blacher RW, Culwell AR, Oltersdorf T et al. Cleavage of amyloid beta peptide during constitutive processing of its precursor. *Science* 1990; 248: 1122–4.

(36) Gandy S, Czernik AJ, Greengard P. Phosphorylation of Alzheimer disease amyloid precursor peptide by protein kinase C and Ca^{2+}/calmodulin-dependent protein kinase II. *Proc Natl Acad Sci USA* 1988; 85: 6218–21.

(37) Buxbaum JD, Gandy SE, Cicchetti P, Ehrlich ME, Czernik AJ, Fracasso RP et al. Processing of Alzheimer beta/A4 amyloid precursor protein: Modulation by agents that regulate protein phosphorylation. *Proc Natl Acad Sci USA* 1990; 87: 6003–6.

(38) Chen WJ, Goldstein JL, Brown MS. NPXY, a sequence often found in cytoplasmic tails, is required for coated pit-mediated internalization of the low density lipoprotein receptor. *J Biol Chem* 1990; 265: 3116–23.

(39) Rosen DR, Martin-Morris L, Luo L, White K. A Drosophila gene encoding a protein resembling the human beta amyloid protein precursor. *Proc Natl Acad Sci USA* 1989; 86: 2478–82.

(40) Martin-Morris LE, White K. The Drosophila transcript encoded by the beta amyloid protein precursor-like gene is restricted to the nervous system. *Development* 1990; 110: 185–95.

(41) Yan YC, Bai Y, Wang L, Miao S, Koide SS. Characterization of a cDNA encoding a human sperm membrane protein related to A4 amyloid protein. *Proc Natl Acad Sci USA* 1990; 87: 2405–8.

(42) Yamaguchi H, Hirai S, Morimatsu M, Shoji M, Ihara Y. A variety of cerebral amyloid deposits in the brains of the Alzheimer-type dementia demonstrated by beta protein immunostaining. *Acta Neuropathol* 1988; 76: 541–9.

(43) Tagliavini F, Giaccone G, Frangione B, Bugiani O. Preamyloid deposits in the cerebral cortex of patients with Alzheimer's disease and nondemented individuals. *Neurosci Lett* 1988; 93: 191–6.

(44) Wisniewski HM, Bancher C, Barcikowska M, Wen GY, Curriew J. Spectrum of morphological appearance of amyloid deposits in Alzheimer's disease. *Acta Neuropathol* 1989; 78: 337–47.

(45) Joachim CL, Morris JH, Selkoe DJ. Diffuse senile plaques occur commonly in the cerebellum in Alzheimer's disease. *Am J Pathol* 1989; 135: 309–19.

(46) Verga L, Frangione B, Tagliavini F, Giaccone G, Migheli A, Bugiani O. Alzheimer patients and Down patients: cerebral preamyloid deposits differ ultrastructurally and histochemically from the amyloid of senile plaques. *Neurosci Lett* 1989; 105: 294–9.

(47) Arai H, Lee VMY, Otvos L, Greenberg BD, Lowery DE, Sharma SK et al. Defined neurofilament, tau, and beta amyloid precursor epitopes distinguish Alzheimer from non-Alzheimer senile plaques. *Proc Natl Acad Sci USA* 1990; 87: 2249–53.

(48) Spillantini MG, Goedert M, Jakes R, Klug A. Different configurational states of beta amyloid and their distributions relative to plaques and tangles in Alzheimer disease. *Proc Natl Acad Sci USA* 1990; 87: 3947–51.

(49) Wattendorff AR, Bots GTAM, Went LN, Endtz LJ. Familial cerebral amyloid angiopathy presenting as recurrent cerebral haemorrhage. *J Neurol Sci* 1982; 55: 121–35.

(50) Van Duinen SG, Castano EM, Prelli F, Bots GTAB, Luyendijk W, Frangione B. Hereditary cerebral hemorrhage with amyloidosis in patients of Dutch origin is related to Alzheimer disease. *Proc Natl Acad Sci USA* 1987; 84: 5991–4.

(51) Van Broeckhoven C, Haan J, Bakker E, Hardy JA, Van Hul W et al. Amyloid beta protein precursor gene and hereditary cerebral hemorrhage with amyloidosis (Dutch). *Science* 1990; 248: 1120–2.

(52) Levy E, Carman MD, Fernandez-Madrid IJ, Power MD, Lieberburg I, Van Duinen SG et al. Mutation of the Alzheimer's disease amyloid gene in hereditary cerebral hemorrhage, Dutch type. *Science* 1990; 248: 1124–6.

(53) Kidd M. Paired helical filaments in electron microscopy of Alzheimer's disease. *Nature* 1963; 197: 192–3.

(54) Gambetti P, Autilio-Gambetti L, Perry G, Scheckel G, Crane RC. Antibodies to

neurofibrillary tangles of Alzheimer's disease raised from human and animal neurofilament fractions. *Lab Invest* 1983; 49: 25–39.

(55) Yen SH, Gaskin F, Fu SM. Neurofibrillary tangles in senile dementia of the Alzheimer type share an antigenic determinant with intermediate filaments of the vimentin class. *Am J Pathol* 1983; 113: 373–81.

(56) Mori H, Kondo J, Ihara Y. Ubiquitin is a component of paired helical filaments in Alzheimer's disease. *Science* 1987; 235: 1641–4.

(57) Perry G, Friedman R, Shaw G, Chau V. Ubiquitin is detected in neurofibrillary tangles and senile plaque neurites of Alzheimer's disease brain. *Proc Natl Acad Sci USA* 1987; 84: 3033–6.

(58) Masters CL, Multhaup G, Simms G, Pottgiesser J, Martins RN, Beyreuther K. Neuronal origin of cerebral amyloid: neurofibrillary tangles of Alzheimer's disease contain the same protein as amyloid plaque cores and blood vessels. *EMBO J* 1985; 4: 2757–63.

(59) Mesulam MM, Moran MA. Cholinesterases within neurofibrillary tangles related to age and Alzheimer's disease. *Ann Neurol* 1987; 22: 223–8.

(60) Brion JP, Passareiro JP, Nunez J, Flament-Durand J. Mise en évidence immunologique de la protéine tau au niveau des lésions de dégénérescence neurofibrillaire de la maladie d'Alzheimer. *Arch. Biol.* 1985; 95: 229–35.

(61) Wood JG, Mirra SS, Pollock NJ, Binder LI. Neurofibrillary tangles of Alzheimer disease share antigenic determinants with the axonal microtubule-associated protein tau. *Proc Natl Acad Sci USA* 1986; 83: 4040–3.

(62) Kosik K, Joachim CL, Selkoe DJ. Microtubule-associated protein tau is a major antigenic component of paired helical filaments in Alzheimer disease. *Proc Natl Acad Sci USA* 1986; 83: 4044–8.

(63) Grundke-Iqbal I, Iqbal K, Quinlan M, Tung YC, Zaidi MS, Wisniewski HM. Microtubule-associated protein tau: a component of Alzheimer paired helical filaments. *J Biol Chem* 1986; 261: 6084–9.

(64) Delacourte A, Défossez A. Alzheimer's disease: Tau proteins, the promoting factors of microtubule assembly are major components of paired helical filaments. *J Neurol Sci* 1986; 76: 173–86.

(65) Kosik KS, Duffy LK, Dowling MM, Abraham C, McCloskey A, Selkoe DJ. Microtubule-associated protein 2: monoclonal antibodies demonstrate the selective incorporation of certain epitopes into Alzheimer neurofibrillary tangles. *Proc Natl Acad Sci USA* 1984; 81: 7941–5.

(66) Crowther RA, Wischik CM. Image reconstruction of the Alzheimer paired helical filament. *EMBO J* 1985; 4: 3661–5.

(67) Wischik CM, Novak M, Edwards PC, Klug A, Tichelaar W, Crowther RA. Structural characterization of the core of the paired helical filament of Alzheimer disease. *Proc Natl Aad Sci USA* 1988; 85: 4884–8.

(68) Wischik CM, Novak M, Thøgersen HC, Edwards PC, Runswick MJ, Jakes R et al. Isolation of a fragment of tau derived from the core of the Alzheimer paired helical filament. *Proc Natl Acad Sci USA* 1988; 85: 4506–10.

(69) Goedert M, Wischik CM, Crowther RA, Walker JE, Klug A. Cloning and sequencing of the cDNA encoding a core protein of the paired helical filament of Alzheimer disease: identification as the microtubule-associated protein tau. *Proc Natl Acad Sci USA* 1988; 85: 4051–5.

(70) Goedert M, Spillantini MG, Potier MC, Ulrich J, Crowther RA. Cloning and sequencing of the cDNA encoding an isoform of microtubule-associated protein tau containing four tandem repeats: Differential expression of tau protein mRNAs in human brain. *EMBO J* 1989; 8: 393–9.

(71) Mori H, Hamada Y, Kawaguchi M, Honda T, Kondo J, Ihara Y. A distinct form of tau is selectively incorporated into Alzheimer's paired helical filaments. *Biochem Biophys Res Commun* 1989; 159: 1221–6.

(72) Ennulat DJ, Liem RKH, Hashim GA, Shelanski ML. Two separate 18 amino acid domains of tau promote the polymerization of tubulin. *J Biol Chem* 1989; 264: 5327–30.

(73) Lee G, Neve RL, Kosik KS. The microtubule-binding domain of tau protein. *Neuron* 1989; 2: 1615–24.

(74) Lewis SA, Wang D, Cowan NJ. Microtubule-associated protein MAP2 shares a microtubule binding motif with tau protein. *Science* 1988; 242: 936–9.

(75) Aizawa H, Emori Y, Murofushi H, Kawasaki H, Sakai H, Suzuki K. Molecular cloning of a ubiquitously distributed microtubule-assocated protein with M_r 190,000. *J Biol Chem* 1990; 265: 13849–55.

(76) Goedert M, Spillantini MG, Jakes R, Rutherford D, Crowther RA. Sequences of multiple isoforms of human microtubule-associated protein tau and their presence in neurofibrillary tangles of Alzheimer's disease. *Neuron* 1989; 3: 519–26.

(77) Lee G, Cowan N, Kirschner M. The primary structure and heterogeneity of tau protein from mouse brain. *Science* 1988; 239: 285–8.

(78) Kanai Y, Takemura R, Oshima T, Morei H, Ihara Y, Yanagisawa M et al. Expression of multiple tau isoforms and microtubule bundle formation in fibroblasts transfected with a single tau cDNA. *J Cell Biol* 1989; 109: 1173–84.

(79) Himmler A, Drechsel D, Kirschner MW, Martin DW. Tau consists of a set of proteins with repeated C-terminal microtubule-binding domains and variable N-terminal domains. *Mol Cell Biol* 1989; 9: 1381–8.

(80) Himmler A. The structure of the bovine tau gene: Alternatively spliced transcripts generate a protein family. *Mol Cell Biol* 1989; 9: 1389–96.

(81) Kondo J, Honda T, Mori H, Hamada Y, Miura R, Ogawara M, Ihara Y. The carboxyl third of tau is tightly bound to paired helical filaments. *Neuron* 1988; 1: 827–34.

(82) Matus A, Bernhardt R, Hugh-Jones T. High molecular weight microtubule-associated proteins are preferentially associated with dendritic microtubules in brain. *Proc Natl Acad Sci USA* 1981; 78: 3010–14.

(83) Binder LI, Frankfurter A, Rebhun LI. The distribution of tau in the mammalian nervous system. *J Cell Biol* 1985; 101: 1371–8.

(84) Papandrikopoulou A, Doll T, Tucker TP, Garner CC, Matus A. Embryonic MAP2 lacks the cross-linking sidearm sequences and dendritic targeting signal of MAP2. *Nature* 1989; 340: 650–2.

(85) Kindler S, Schulz B, Goedert M, Garner CC. Molecular structure of microtubule-associated protein 2b and 2c from rat brain. *J Biol Chem* 1990; 265: 19679–84.

(86) Garner CC, Tucker RP, Matus A. Selective localization of messenger RNA for cytoskeletal protein MAP2 in dendrites. *Nature* 1988; 336: 674–7.

(87) Okabe S, Hirokawa N. Rapid turnover of microtubule-associated protein MAP2 in the axon revealed by microinjection of biotinylated MAP2 into cultured neurons. *Proc Natl Acad Sci USA* 1989; 86: 4127–31.

(88) Hirokawa N, Okabe S. Selective stabilization of microinjected microtubule-associated protein 2 (MAP2) in dendrites and tau in the axon of the neuronal cytoskeleton. *J Cell Biol* 1989; 109: 78a.

(89) Goedert M, Jakes R. Expression of separate isoforms of human tau protein: correlation with the tau pattern in brain and effects on tubulin polymerization. *EMBO J* 1990; 9: 4225–30.

(90) Steinert B, Mandelkow EM, Biernat J, Gustke N, Meyer HE, Schmidt B et al. Phosphorylation of microtubule-associated protein tau: Identification of the site for Ca^{2+}/calmodulin-dependent kinase and relationship with tau phosphorylation in Alzheimer tangles. *EMBO J* 1990; 9: 3539–44.

(91) Baudier J, Cole RD. Phosphorylation of tau proteins to a state like that in Alzheimer's brain is catalyzed by a calcium/calmodulin-dependent kinase and modulated by phospholipids. *J Biol Chem* 1987; 262: 17577–83.

(92) Lindwall G, Cole RD. Phosphorylation affects the ability of tau protein to promote microtubule assembly. *J Biol Chem* 1984; 259: 5301–5.

(93) Grundke-Iqbal I, Iqbal K, Tung YC, Quinlan M, Wisniewski HM, Binder U. Abnormal phosphorylation of the microtubule-associated protein tau in Alzheimer cytoskeletal pathology. *Proc Natl Acad Sci USA* 1986; 83: 4913–17.

(94) Flament S, Delacourte A, Hémon B, Défossez A. Characterization of two pathological tau protein variants in Alzheimer brain cortices. *J Neurol Sci* 1989; 92: 133–41.

(95) Flament S, Delacourte A, Delaère P, Duyckaerts C, Hauw JJ. Correlation between microscopical changes and Tau 64 and 69 biochemical detection in senile dementia of the Alzheimer type. *Acta Neuropathol* 1990; 80: 212–15.

(96) Selkoe DJ, Ihara Y, Salazar FJ. Alzheimer's disease: insolubility of partially purified paired helical filaments in sodium dodecyl sulphate and urea. *Science* 1982; 215: 1243–5.

(97) Greenberg SG, Davies P. A preparation of Alzheimer paired helical filaments that displays distinct tau proteins by polyacrylamide gel electrophoresis. *Proc Natl Acad Sci USA* 1990; 87: 5827–31.

(98) Spillantini MG, Goedert M, Jakes R, Klug A. Topographical relationship between beta-amyloid and tau protein epitopes in tangle-bearing cells in Alzheimer disease. *Proc Natl Acad Sci USA* 1990; 87: 3952–6.

Neurochemical studies of cortical and subcortical dementias

A J CROSS

Introduction

The differentiation of subcortical and cortical dementias was formalized by Albert[1] who used the term 'subcortical dementia' to describe the cognitive deficits of progressive supranuclear palsy. Since that time, the concept has been applied extensively, especially in contrasting the cognitive impairments which are frequently associated with disorders of motor function (i.e. Parkinson's disease and Huntington's chorea (HC)) to those of Alzheimer-type dementia (ATD) and Pick's disease (PD). Despite providing a useful framework for classifying these disorders, the concept has remained controversial and has stimulated considerable debate[2-5].

The distinctions between cortical and subcortical dementias were made primarily on neuropsychological grounds.[2] Thus cortical dementias are associated with focal cortical dysfunction such as aphasia, agnosia and amnesia. Subcortical dementias are characterized by bradyphrenia, visuospatial disorder and mood disturbance. These distinctions are summarized in Table 1. It is clear, however, that there is considerable overlap between the clinical features of ATD, PD and HC.

Consideration of the distribution of the neuropathological lesions in dementing illnesses has not provided an unequivocal distinction between cortical and subcortical dementias. Thus several of the diseases may display similar neuropathological lesions (e.g. neurofibrillary tangles in progressive supranuclear palsy, Lewy bodies in dementia) and indeed there may be considerable overlap in the anatomical distribution of the lesions. It is quite possible, therefore, that consideration of the neurochemical changes present in cortical and subcortical dementias may further complicate any distinctions. However, it is to be hoped that by comparing neurochemical changes in diseases which fall broadly into the classification of cortical or subcortical

All correspondence to: Dr AJ Cross, Astra Neuroscience Research Unit, 1 Wakefield Street, London WC1N 1PJ, UK.

Cambridge Medical Reviews: Neurobiology and Psychiatry Volume 1
© Cambridge University Press

Table 1. *The distinction between cortical and subcortical dementia.*

Characteristic	Subcortical	Cortical
Language	No aphasia	Aphasia
Memory	Mild impairment	Amnesia
Cognition	Impaired	Severely impaired (agnosia, aphasia)
Mood	Affective disorder common	Normal
Motor function	Impaired	Normal

Modified from Brown & Marsden[2].

dementia, that some correlations can be made with the clinical features which distinguish these diseases.

It has recently become clear that several 'atypical' dementing illnesses may be more prevalent than previously supposed. The most relevant of these to the present discussion are diffuse Lewy body dementia[6] and senile dementia of Lewy body type[7], as some neurochemical data are available. It is not the purpose of the present review to describe in detail the neurochemical changes associated with these diseases. However, the possibility that these atypical dementias represent distinct disease entities, and the subsequent neurochemical studies have provided added insight to the distinction between cortical and subcortical dementias.

Neurochemical changes in Alzheimer-type dementia
In the neocortex of ATD patients, a number of neurochemical changes have been observed which are consistent with degeneration of the terminals of ascending neurones. The most severely affected system appears to be the cholinergic system. The loss of the marker enzyme choline acetyltransferase (ChAT) occurs throughout the neo- and archicortex, and is found in patients with relatively mild neuropathological changes[8-10]. Evidence from biopsy samples suggests that ChAT activity and acetylcholine synthesis are lost within 3–4 years of the onset of symptoms[11].

Other ascending neurones may also be involved, although to a lesser extent (Fig. 1). In the temporal lobe, serotonergic terminals are reduced to almost the same extent as cholinergic terminals[12,13], although this is not the case in other brain regions. Noradrenergic terminals are also lost, although to a lesser extent[14,15]. There is now a considerable body of evidence to suggest that these ascending neurones undergo a process of retrograde degeneration following primary damage in the cortex. This evidence is briefly summarized in Table 2.

Within the neocortex and archicortex it has been possible to demonstrate that selective neurochemical changes occur in ATD[16,17], although these may

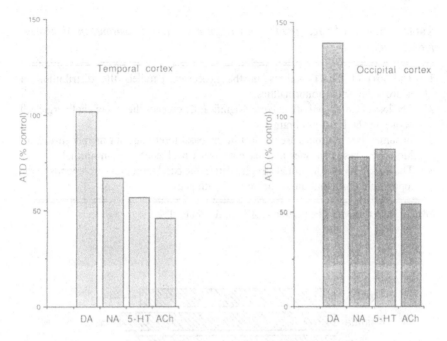

Fig. 1. Cortical afferents in Alzheimer-type dementia. Neurochemical markers were as follows: dopamine (DA) neurones: HVA concentration, noradrenaline (NA): dopamine-β-hydroxylase activity, serotonin (5-HT): serotonin concentrations, acetylcholine (ACh): choline acetyltransferase activity. Note equivalent loss of ACh in both temporal and occipital cortex, whilst 5-HT is lost significantly only in temporal cortex. (Data[12, 15] and from unpublished observations.)

not be apparent in the most severely affected patients with advanced cerebral degeneration[18]. Neurofibrillary tangles are present predominantly in the pyramidal neurones of layers III and V of the neocortex[19]. These neurones form intrinsic cortical and descending connections respectively, and most probably use an excitatory amino acid (EAA) as transmitter[20,21]. Neurochemical markers of EAA containing neurones are reduced in ATD[22,23], lending strong support to the suggestion that pyramidal neurones degenerate[24,25]. The other major cortical neurotransmitter, GABA, is not reduced in mild to moderately affected patients. In severely affected patients, neurochemical markers of GABA neurones may be reduced[26], and particularly those GABA neurones which also contain somatostatin[27]. Selective changes are also observed in neurotransmitter receptors (Fig. 2), in this case the 5-HT$_2$ receptor is markedly reduced whilst other receptors remain unchanged[28]. 5-HT$_2$ receptors are not concentrated on the terminals of ascending cholinergic neurones. However, the distribution of the reduction of 5-HT$_2$ receptors in

A J Cross

Table 2. *Evidence for retrograde degeneration of cholinergic neurones in Alzheimer-type dementia*

1. The loss of ChAT activity in the neocortex parallels the distribution of neuropathological abnormalities.
2. The loss of ChAT activity in cortex significantly exceeds the loss of cholinergic cell bodies in the basal forebrain.
3. In some cases neurones are not lost in the basal forebrain, but merely shrunken. Moreover these neurones may have a lower ChAT content than normal.
4. The distribution of neuronal atrophy within the basal forebrain corresponds to the topographic distribution of the cortical pathology.

Adapted from Candy et al[35], Pearson et al[19] and Arendt et al[30].

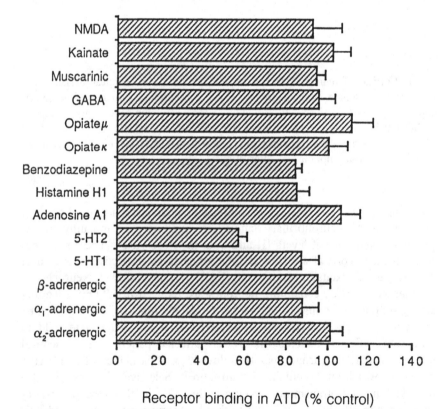

Receptor binding in ATD (% control)

Fig. 2. Neurotransmitter receptor binding sites in ATD. Data[23, 28]. Note large reduction in 5-HT$_2$ receptors with little change in other receptor binding sites.

ATD closely parallels the distribution of cortical pathological change[29]. The changes in markers of both EAA neurones and 5-HT$_2$ receptors correlate with the severity of cortical pathology.

It has been possible to make a number of clinical and pathological correlations in ATD. The loss of cortical cholinergic terminals correlates with the degree of dementia[8]. Other ascending neurotransmitter systems which are affected in ATD may be unrelated to overall measures of the severity of dementia. In particular, markers of serotonergic and noradrenergic terminals do not correlate with dementia ratings[31].

The densities of senile plaques and neurofibrillary tangles in neocortex also correlate with the severity of dementia[32,33]. These correlations are stronger for neurofibrillary tangle densities, suggesting an involvement of pyramidal neurones. This suggestion is further emphasized by the correlations between loss or histologic abnormality of these cells and the severity of dementia. Thus the dementia of Alzheimer's disease seems to relate to dysfunction of both ascending cholinergic neurones and cortical pyramidal neurones.

Neurochemical changes in Parkinson's disease
It has become clear that many neurotransmitter systems other than dopamine are involved in the pathophysiology of Parkinson's disease (PD)[34]. Within the neocortex, ChAT activity is markedly reduced. In this case the loss of cortical ChAT activity as accompanied by an equivalent loss of cholinergic cell bodies in the basal forebrain[35,36]. Other ascending systems are also involved. Thus reductions in serotonin and noradrenaline have been noted in PD[34]; however, losses of these neurotransmitters do not correlate with the presence of dementia[37,38] (Fig. 3).

Neurochemical markers of intrinsic cortical neurones are not generally reduced in the absence of consistent Alzheimer-type changes. Thus neurochemical markers of glutamate neurones (Fig. 4) and 5-HT$_2$ receptors are unchanged in PD[39,40]. In severely demented patients, cortical concentrations of somatostatin may be reduced; however, in this situation it is difficult to exclude the possibility of coincidental Alzheimer's disease. In none of these cases does the neurochemical index correlate with the presence of dementia[41].

Several studies suggest that the loss of cortical ChAT activity in PD corresponds to the presence of dementia[42,43]. It should, however, be noted that apparently non-demented Parkinson's disease patients have some loss of cortical ChAT activity. Whilst cortical dopamine concentrations are not lower in PD patients with dementia, it has been suggested that dementia is a late development in the course of the disease[44]. In this regard, it should be noted that striatal dopamine concentrations are lower in demented PD patients compared to patients without dementia[45].

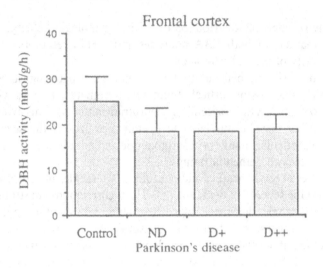

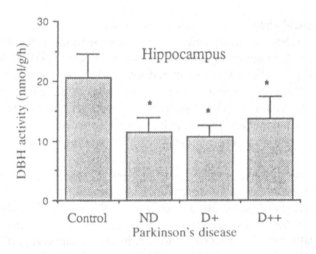

Fig. 3. Dopamine-β-hydroxylase activity in Parkinson's disease (PD). Whilst dopamine-β-hydroxylase activity is reduced in the hippocampus of ATD and PD patients, there is no relationship to the presence of dementia in the PD patients. ND: non-demented patients; D+: moderate dementia; D++: severe dementia. *$P<0.05$. Data from Allen et al[56].

Other dementing illnesses

In progressive supranuclear palsy (PSP), a marked striatal dopaminergic deficit is observed, comparable to that of PD. In contrast to PD, this does not correlate with the presence of dementia[46]. Whilst cortical and mesolimbic

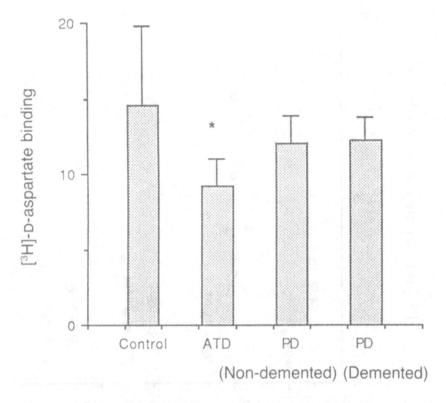

Fig. 4. [³H]-D-aspartic acid binding in ATD and PD cortex. Whilst a significant reduction is observed in ATD, no change is present in Parkinson's disease patients with or without dementia. *$P<0.05$. From Cross et al[40].

dopaminergic systems remain intact in PSP, ascending cholinergic systems may degenerate[47]. It has been proposed that the cholinergic deficit in PSP may relate to the intellectual deterioration[48], although this may not always be the case[49]. The loss of cortical ChAT activity is certainly not as extensive as in ATD or PD.

Cortical Lewy bodies are found in a number of dementing illnesses, including PD, Hallervorden–Spatz disease and diffuse Lewy body dementia (DLBD). The distinction between PD and DLBD has been questioned[4] and there have been no specific neurochemical studies. However, it has recently become clear that a significant proportion of patients with dementia in old age are characterized neuropathologically by the presence of cortical senile plaques and Lewy bodies and minimal neurofibrillary tangle formation[7,50]. It has been proposed[7] that this may represent a distinct disease, termed senile dementia of Lewy body type (SDLT). Neurochemical studies have demonstrated a loss of cortical ChAT activity equivalent to that of ATD, which

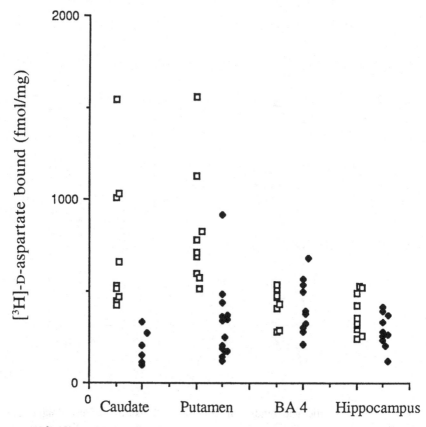

Fig. 5. [³H]-D-aspartic acid binding in Huntington's disease. Binding is significantly reduced in candate nucleus and putamen, and is unchanged in frontal (BA4) cortex and hippocampus. □: control subjects, ◆: Huntington's disease patients. From Cross et al[52].

correlated with the severity of dementia[50]. Cell loss in the locus coeruleus and substantia nigra did not correlate with the degree of dementia[50].

In addition to the involvement of the basal ganglia in Huntington's chorea, there is some evidence that the cerebral cortex is also involved. Neurochemical studies have shown that markers of the terminals of cortical–striatal neurones are reduced in HC[51,52] (Fig. 5), and that this loss is greatest in severely demented HC patients[53]. Whilst cortical cholinergic systems remain intact, several studies have shown that hippocampal serotonergic and cholinergic systems may be disrupted[52,53]. In the case of the hippocampal cholinergic system, this does not relate to the presence of dementia[53].

Clinical correlates

From the studies outlined above it is clear that two broad conclusions can be drawn.

1. A cortical cholinergic deficit is present in many dementing illnesses, previously classified as either cortical (i.e. ATD, Pick's disease) or subcortical (i.e. PD, PSP).
2. Neurochemical markers of cortical pyramidal neurones are also reduced in some dementing illnesses, again these have been classified as either cortical (i.e. ATD) or subcortical (i.e. HC).

On this basis, a simple classification of cortical/subcortical dementia would not seem to be supported by neurochemical studies. This is hardly surprising as the neurotransmitter systems implicated in the pathology of these diseases are involved in either the ascending (acetylcholine) or descending (EAA) connections of the cerebral cortex (Table 3). Despite this, it is possible to draw some support for the concept of subcortical dementia. In SDLT, the clinical picture may be closer to that of a subcortical dementia rather than cortical dementia. As noted by Perry et al[50], these symptoms of SDLT are reminiscent of those resulting from anticholinergic intake. The reduction in cortical ChAT activity is equivalent to that of Parkinson's disease patients with dementia, and greater than that noted in ATD. One might therefore speculate that the cognitive impairment of subcortical dementia relates to the loss of cholinergic input to the cortex. This is supported by the observation that in PSP, there is also a loss of cortical cholinergic terminals. In ATD the 'subcortical cholinergic deficit' is present, but it is complicated by the changes present in cortical pyramidal neurones. The loss of cortical pyramidal neurones is greatest in the association areas of the temporal–parietal regions. It is these regions which are frequently associated with the cortical signs of ATD, i.e. aphasia, apraxia and agnosia. The involvement of the ascending cholinergic system in Pick's disease is less clear, and it may well be that cortical changes predominate. In ATD there is evidence for retrograde degeneration of cholinergic neurones. There is, however, no direct evidence to link the pathological changes in neocortical neurones with cholinergic degeneration. In Parkinson's disease it would seem more likely that anterograde degeneration of cholinergic neurones occurs.

This discussion is of course an oversimplification. No account has been taken of changes outside the cerebral cortex and basal ganglia. Of particular relevance is the hippocampus, which is intimately involved in specific memory processes. In ATD the involvement of the hippocampal cholinergic system, and intrinsic EAA neurones are well documented[54]. It would be surprising if these changes did not contribute significantly to the clinical features of the disease. In addition, the simple classification outlined above does not take account of Huntington's chorea. The role of the basal forebrain cholinergic system in HC is minimal (although hippocampal ChAT is

Table 3. *Cortical neurotransmitter changes in dementing illnesses*

		Alzheimer-type dementia	Parkinson's disease	Huntington's chorea
Ascending neurones	Acetylcholine	Reduced[a]	Reduced[a]	Unchanged
	5-hydroxytryptamine	Reduced	Reduced	Unchanged
	Dopamine	Unchanged	Reduced	Unchanged
	Noradrenaline	Reduced	Reduced	Unchanged
Cortical neurones	Excitatory amino acid	Reduced[a]	Unchanged	Reduced[a]
	5-HT$_2$ receptor	Reduced	Unchanged	Unchanged
	Somatostatin	Reduced (?)	Reduced (?)	Unchanged
	GABA	Unchanged	Unchanged	Reduced

[a] Significant relationship to the presence of dementia.

reduced) whereas the cortico-striatal glutamatergic pathway is involved, consistent with a loss of cortical glutamatergic neurones. On this basis one would classify HC as a 'cortical' dementia.

Despite these reservations, it is possible that these findings have some relevance to the treatment of dementing illnesses. The 'cholinergic theory' of memory impairment in ATD has led to the development of many cholinergic compounds for the possible treatment of dementia. An improvement in some patients with clinically diagnosed ATD has been observed following treatment with the cholinesterase inhibitor tacrine[55]. It is clear, however, that only a proportion of ATD patients are responsive to such treatment. One might predict that those patients with a more predominant cholinergic deficit (i.e. SDLT and PD) would be more responsive than those with an additional cortical deficit such as in ATD. Indeed it would be ironic if a drug treatment devised for a cortical dementia was found to be more effective for the treatment of subcortical dementia.

References

(1) Albert ML, Feldman RG, Willis AL. The 'subcortical dementia' of progressive supranuclear palsy. *J Neurol, Neurosurg Psychiat* 1974; 37: 121–30.
(2) Brown RG, Marsden CD. 'Subcortical dementia': the neuropsychological evidence. *Neuroscience* (1988); 25: 363–87.
(3) Whitehouse PJ. The concept of subcortical and cortical dementia: another look. *Ann Neurol* 1986; 19: 1–6.
(4) Gibb WRG. Dementia and Parkinson's disease. *Br J Psychiat* 1989; 154: 596–614.
(5) Cunningham JL. Subcortical dementia: neuropsychology, neuropsychiatry and pathophysiology. *Br J Psychiat* 1986; 149: 682–7.
(6) Ikeda K, Mori A, Bode G. Progressive dementia with 'diffuse Lewy-type inclu-

sions' in cerebral cortex. A case report. *Arch Psychiat Nervenks* 1980; 228: 243–8.

(7) Perry RM, Irving D, Blessed G, Perry EK, Smith CJ, Fairburn AF. Dementia in old age: identification of a clinically and pathologically distinct disease entity. *Adv Neurol* 1990; 51: 41–6.

(8) Perry EK, Tomlinson BE, Blessed G, Bergmann K, Gibson PH, Perry RH. Correlation of cholinergic abnormalities with senile plaques and mental test scores in senile dementia. *Br Med J* 1978; ii: 1457–9.

(9) Bowen DM, Spillane JA, Curzon G et al. Accelerated ageing or selective or selective neuronal loss as an important cause of dementia. *Lancet* 1979; i: 11–4.

(10) Davies P. Neurotransmitter-related enzymes in senile dementia of the Alzheimer type. *Brain Res* 1979; 171: 319–27.

(11) Bowen DM, Allen SJ, Benton JS et al. Biochemical assessment of serotonergic and cholinergic dysfunction and cerebral atrophy in Alzheimer's disease. *J Neurochem* 1983; 43: 266–78.

(12) Cross AJ, Crow TJ, Johnson JA et al. Monoamine metabolism in senile dementia of Alzheimer-type. *J Neurol Sci* 1983; 60: 383–92.

(13) Palmer AM, Willcock GK, Esiri MM, Francis PT, Bowen DM. Monoaminergic innervation of frontal and temporal lobe in Alzheimer's disease. *Brain Res* 1987; 401: 231–40.

(14) Adolfsson R, Gottfries CG, Roos BE, Winblad B. Changes in brain catecholamines in patients with dementia of Alzheimer type. *Br J Psychiat* 1979; 135: 216–23.

(15) Cross AJ, Crow TJ, Perry EK, Perry RH, Blessed G, Tomlinson BE. Reduced dopamine-β-hydroxylase activity in Alzheimer's disease. *Br Med J* 1981; 282: 93–4.

(16) Cross AJ, Crow TJ, Peters TJ. Cortical neurochemistry in Alzheimer-type dementia. *Prog Brain Res* 1986; 70: 153–69.

(17) Bowen DM, Davison AN. Biochemical studies of nerve cells and energy metabolism in Alzheimer's disease. *Br Med Bull* 1986; 42: 75–80.

(18) Hubbard BM, Anderson JM. A quantitative study of cerebral atrophy in old age and senile dementia. *J Neurol Sci* 1981; 50: 135–45.

(19) Pearson RCA, Esiri MM, Hiorns MW, Wilcock GK, Powell TPS. Anatomical correlates of the distribution of the pathological changes in the neocortex in Alzheimer's disease. *Proc Natl Acad Sci USA* 1988; 82: 4531–6.

(20) Fonnum F. Glutamate – a neurotransmitter in mammalian brain. *J Neurochem* 1984; 42: 1–11.

(21) Fagg GE, Foster AC. Amino acid neurotransmitters and their pathways in the mammalian central nervous system. *Neuroscience* 1983; 9: 707–19.

(22) Palmer AM, Proctor AW, Stratmann GC, Bowen DM. Excitatory amino acid – releasing and cholinergic neurones in Alzheimer's disease. *Neurosci Lett* 1986; 66: 199–204.

(23) Simpson MDC, Royston MC, Deakin JFW, Cross AJ, Mann DMA, Slater P. Regional changes in [^{3}H]-d-aspartate binding and [^{3}H]-TCP binding sites in Alzheimers disease brains. *Brain Res* 1988: 76–82.

(24) Pearce BR, Palmer AM, Bowen DM, Wilcock GK, Esiri MM, Davison AN.

Neurotransmitter dysfunction and atrophy of the caudate nucleus in Alzheimers disease. *Neurochem Pathol* 1984; 2: 221–32.

(25) Cross AJ, Crow TJ, Ferrier IN, Johnson JA, Markakis D. Striatal dopamine receptors in Alzheimer-type dementia. *Neurosci Lett* 1984; 52: 1–6.

(26) Rossor MN, Iversen LL, Reynolds GP, Mountjoy CQ, Roth M. Neurochemical characteristics of early and late onset types of Alzheimer's disease. *Br Med J* 1984; 288: 961–4.

(27) Davies P, Katzman R, Terry RD. Reduced somatostatin-like immunoreactivity in cerebral cortex of Alzheimer disease and senile dementia. *Nature* 1980; 288: 279–80.

(28) Cross AJ, Crow TJ, Ferrier IN, Johnson JA. The selectivity of the reduction of serotonin S2 receptors in Alzheimer-type dementia. *Neurobiol Aging* 1986; 7: 3–12.

(29) Proctor AW, Lowe SL, Palmer AM et al. Topographical distribution of neurochemical changes in Alzheimer's disease. *J Neurol Sci* 1988; 84: 125–40.

(30) Arendt T, Bigl V, Tennstedt A, Arendt A. Neuronal loss in different parts of the nucleus basalis is related to neuritic plaque formation in cortical target areas in Alzheimers disease. *Neuroscience* 1985; 14: 1–14.

(31) Cross AJ. Serotonin in neurodegenerative disorders. In: Osborne NN, Hamon M, eds. *Neuronal serotonin*. Chichester: John Wiley, 1988: 231–53.

(32) Wilcock GK, Esiri MM. Plaques tangles and dementia. A quantitative study. *J Neurol Sci* 1982; 56: 343–56.

(33) Mann DMA. The neuropathology of Alzheimers disease: a review with pathogenic, aetiological and therapeutic considerations. *Mech Aging Dev* 1985; 31: 213–35.

(34) Hornykiewicz O. Parkinson's disease: from brain homogenate to treatment. *Fed Proc* 1973; 32: 183–90.

(35) Candy JM, Perry RH, Perry EK et al. Pathological changes in the nucleus of Meynert in Alzheimer's and Parkinson's disease. *J Neurol Sci* 1983a; 54: 277–89.

(36) Gaspar P, Gray F. Dementia in idiopathic Parkinson's disease. A neuropathological study of 32 cases. *Acta Neuropath* 1984; 64: 43–52.

(37) Cash R, Dennis TL, Heureux R et al. Parkinson's disease and dementia: norepinephrine and dopamine in locus coeruleus. *Neurology* 1989; 37: 42–6.

(38) Scatton B, Javoy-Agid F, Rouquier L, Dubois B, Agid Y. Reduction of cortical dopamine, noradrenaline, serotonin and their metabolites in Parkinsons disease. *Brain Res* 1983; 321–3.

(39) Perry EK, Perry RM, Candy JM et al. Cortical serotonin S2 receptors binding abnormalities in patients with Alzheimer's disease: comparisons with Parkinson's disease. *Neurosci Lett* 1984; 51: 353–7.

(40) Cross AJ, Slater P, Simpson M et al. Sodium dependent [^{3}H]-d-aspartate binding in cerebral cortex in patients with Alzheimer's and Parkinson's disease. *Neurosci Lett* 1987; 79: 213–17.

(41) Epelbaum J, Ruberg M, Moyse E et al. Somatostatin and dementia in Parkinson disease. *Brain Res* 1983; 278: 376–9.

(42) Ruberg M, Ploska A, Javoy-Agid F et al. Muscarinic binding and choline

acetyltransferase activity in parkinsonian subjects with reference to dementia. *Brain Res* 232: 129–39.

(43) Perry EK, Curtis M, Dick DJ et al. Cholinergic correlates and cognitive impairment in Parkinson's disease: comparisons with Alzheimer's disease. *J Neurol Neurosurg Psychiat* 1985; 48: 413–21.

(44) Ball MJ. The morphological basis of dementia in Parkinson's disease. *Can J Neurol Sci* 1984; 11: 180–4.

(45) Scatton B, Rouquier L, Javoy-Agid F et al. Dopamine deficiency in the cerebral cortex in Parkinson disease. *Neurology* 1982; 32: 1039–40.

(46) Bokobza B, Ruberg M, Scatton B et al. [³H]-spiperone binding, dopamine and HVA concentrations in Parkinson's disease and supranuclear palsy. *Eur J Pharmacol* 1984; 99: 167–75.

(47) Ruberg M, Javoy-Agid F, Hirsch E et al. Dopaminergic and cholinergic lesions in progressive supranuclear palsy. *Ann Neurol* 1985; 18: 523–9.

(48) Tagliavia F, Pilleri G, Bociras C, Constantinidis J. The basal nucleus of Meynert in patients with progressive supranuclear palsy. *Neurosci Lett* 1984; 44: 37–42.

(49) Kish SJ, Chang LJ, Mirchardi L, Shannak K, Hornykiewicz O. Progressive supranuclear palsy: relationship between extrapyramidal disturbances, dementia, and brain neurotransmitter markers. *Ann Neurol* 1985: 530–6.

(50) Perry RM, Irving D, Blessed G, Perry EK, Fairburn AF. Clinically and neuropathologically distinct form of dementia in the elderly. *Lancet* 1989; i: 166.

(51) Cross AJ, Rossor MN. Dopamine D1 and D2 receptors in Huntington's disease. *Eur J Pharmacol* 1983; 88: 223–9.

(52) Cross AJ, Slater P, Reynolds GP. Reduced high-affinity glutamate uptake sites in the brains of patients with Huntington's disease. *Neurosci Lett* 1986; 67: 198–202.

(53) Reynolds GP, Pearson SJ, Heathfield WG. Dementia in Huntington's disease is associated with neurochemical deficits in the candate nucleus, not the cerebral cortex. *Neurosci Lett* 1990; 113: 95–100.

(54) Hyman BT, Van Hoesen GW, Damasio AR, Barnes CL. Alzheimer's disease: cell-specific pathology isolates the hippocampus formation. *Science* 1984; 225: 1168–70.

(55) Summers WK, Majorski LV, Marsh GM, Tachiki K, Kling A. Oral tetrahydroaminoacridine in long-term treatment of senile dementia, Alzheimer type. *N Engl J Med* 1986; 315: 1241–5.

(56) Allen JN, Cross AJ, Crow TJ, Javoy-Agid F, Agid Y, Bloom SR. Dissociation of neuropeptide Y and somatostatin in Parkinson's disease. *Brain Res* 1985; 337: 197–200.

Subcortical dementia: defining a clinical syndrome

S FLEMINGER

Introduction

This review will discuss some of the methods that have been used to attempt to define a syndrome of dementia resulting from damage to subcortical structures. The distinction between the cortical and subcortical dementias on the basis of neuropathology and neurochemistry is discussed elsewhere in this volume (AJ Cross).

Is it possible to dissect out a clinical syndrome of subcortical dementia from the varied presentation of the archetypal cortical dementia, Alzheimer's disease? What corroborative evidence is there for the validity of the concept of subcortical dementia? What are the methodological issues that one should be aware of when assessing attempts to make such a distinction?

To paraphrase Kendell[1], discussing the role of diagnosis in psychiatry, there are 3 aspects to every dementia syndrome which is secondary to an identified disease, e.g. the dementia of Huntington's disease:

1. those that are shared with all dementias;
2. those that are shared with some, but not all, dementias;
3. those that are unique to that dementia syndrome.

The value of the classification 'subcortical dementia' depends on the size of the second category compared with the other two. What is the relative preponderance of attributes of the dementia of Huntington's disease that are common to all dementias (1), or are singular to Huntington's disease (3), compared with those that are common only to the subcortical dementias (2)?

A historical perspective

The term subcortical dementia was introduced by Albert and colleagues[12] in a paper which addressed the pattern of cognitive and behavioural impairments seen in patients with progressive supranuclear palsy (PSNP). They compared

All correspondence to: Dr S Fleminger, Institute of Psychiatry, De Crespigny Park, Denmark Hill, London SE5 8AF.

Cambridge Medical Reviews: Neurobiology and Psychiatry Volume 1
© Cambridge University Press

their observations of these patients with descriptions in the literature of the dementia produced by other diseases with prominent bilateral subcortical grey matter involvement, in particular Wilson's disease and thalamic degenerations. They concluded that the mental symptoms produced by all these subcortical disease were very similar. They resulted in a dementia of a characteristic pattern, that is distinct from that seen in Alzheimer's disease:

1. Forgetfulness. This they contrasted with the memory loss seen in Alzheimer's disease, and suggested was due to an attentional/retrieval deficit.
2. A slowing of thought processes; bradyphrenia. Characteristically, patients with subcortical dementia will get the correct answer if given long enough to answer. It is therefore important to look at whether tests have a time limit.
3. Emotional or personality changes. Occur relatively early in the course of the subcortical dementias and depression and apathy are particularly prominent.
4. Impaired ability to manipulate acquired knowledge. They are easily muddled and have difficulty making use of information to solve problems. Cognitive tasks that they are familiar with may also be performed poorly.
5. Absence of 'cortical' signs: Aphasia, apraxia and agnosia. There is good evidence from studies of brain lesions that these disorders result from focal damage localized to the cerebral cortex. This is corroborated by their relative absence in the subcortical dementias.

At about the same time, it was reported that the dementia in patients with Huntington's chorea had certain characteristics that were similar to those described by Albert et al. (1974). Huntington's chorea may be regarded as a founder member of the list of diseases producing subcortical dementia.

Albert et al. noted in their review that these subcortical dementias looked rather like the dementia that may be observed following bifrontal disease. Albert (1978) has more recently suggested that fronto-subcortical dementia might be a better label for the syndrome.

Over the last few years, the syndrome of subcortical dementia has received considerable attention. The list of diseases that may result in the syndrome of subcortical dementias is growing; recent additions are AIDS dementia[3], the dementia that may be seen in patients with multiple sclerosis[4] and periventricular white matter disease that may be found in association with cerebrovascular disease[5]. Rather more controversial are suggestions that the mental slowing of depression[6] or the normal elderly[7] should be included in the subcortical dementia syndrome.

Recently Filley et al.[8] have proposed that the subcortical dementias themselves be classified into those with and without white matter involvement;

multiple sclerosis, AIDS dementia and leukoaraiosis[9] resulting in white matter dementias. The neuropsychological impairments seen in two divers with decompression sickness[10] associated with periventricular white matter lesions suggested that it should also be added to any comprehensive list of white matter dementias.

In addition, there has been a temptation to expand the list of neuropsychological disturbances that are to be regarded as typically seen in subcortical dementias. In particular, some authors now regard visuo-spatial dysfunction as part of the syndrome of subcortical dementia[11].

The clinical evidence

There can be little doubt that in certain patients with subcortical disease the clinical picture is very similar to that described in some detail in Albert et al.'s paper.[12] An example of this would be patients with bilateral basal ganglia lesions who tend to show prominent apathy, depression and psychomotor slowing[13–15]. However, because of individual differences identical disease processes may present with different clinical pictures. Lishman[16] notes that 'the impact of chronic diffuse brain disease is not entirely unaffected by features specific to the individual'. The clinical presentations of patients with Alzheimer's disease are heterogeneous; some may present with an isolated memory disturbance, others with personality change, others with an aphasia.

No study has clearly documented that the mental symptoms and behaviour disturbance, excluding those that are directly attributable to neuropsychological impairments, observed in patients with subcortical dementias are different in type or degree from those found in patients with Alzheimer's disease. It seems unlikely that such a study would be successful. For example, depression, regarded as being particularly associated with subcortical dementias, is observed in 20%–40% of patients with Alzheimer's disease[17,18]. Lishman[16] notes that the early stages of Alzheimer's disease are characterized by 'failing memory, muddled inefficiency in the tasks of everyday life, and spatial disorientation. Disturbances of mood may be prominent. . . . Others . . . have stressed aspontaneity, and apathy from the early stages'. These mental symptoms are noteworthy for their similarity to those described as characteristic of subcortical dementia.

EEG studies

Striano et al.[19] propose that the standard EEG may be a useful tool for distinguishing subcortical dementias from cortical. This conclusion is based on their review of the literature and a study comparing the EEGs of patients with Alzheimer's disease with those with multi-infarct dementia. Patients with multi-infarct dementia showed relatively less background slowing of the EEG. They suggested that this finding was compatible with ther review, in that patients with cortical dementia tend to show more slowing of the EEG than is seen in those with subcortical dementias. However, one paper that they quote in support of this conclusion failed in fact to show any difference between the EEGs of demented patients with PSNP compared to those with cortical atrophy[20] (presumably resulting from Alzheimer's disease). In both groups of patients, with predominantly mild to moderate dementia, the majority of patients had EEGs that were regarded as being within normal limits. It seems unlikely, therefore, that conventional EEG will provide useful discrimination between subcortical and cortical dementias.

Evoked potential studies may be more successful in this endeavour. Goodin and Aminoff[21] have found that a delayed N1 potential in the auditory evoked potential was common to patients with dementia with either Huntington's or Parkinson's disease. Patients with Alzheimer's disease showed normal latency N1 potentials. All demented patients showed delay of the N2 and P3 potentials.

Cerebral blood flow and metabolism studies

Salmon & Frank[22] have reviewed the literature on the changes that are observed in cerebral blood flow and metabolism in the various cortical and subcortical dementias.

In Alzheimer's disease there tends to be reductions in cerebral blood flow, associated with reduced cerebral metabolism, over the whole cortex but particularly involving temporal and parietal association cortex. Diseases that result in subcortical dementias may, or may not, produce significant reductions in cortical blood flow, again associated with hypometabolism; where present the reduction may show a frontal predominance.

However, it is clear from the study of the patterns of disturbance of cerebral metabolism found in the various dementias that there are as many differences between the various subcortical dementias as there are differences between the subcortical and cortical dementias. In Huntington's disease there is little, if any, involvement of cortical metabolism despite early hypometabolism in the basal ganglia[23]. Indeed, Weinberger et al.[24] found an *increase* in frontal regional cerebral blood flow in Huntington's disease while the patients were performing the Wisconsin Card Sorting test over and above that seen in control subjects. On the other hand, in PSNP, there is fairly selective hypometabolism in the frontal cortex[25-27].

In Parkinson's disease, no consistent picture has emerged. The pattern of cortical involvement may be similar to that observed in Alzheimer's disease[23]. Some studies have failed to show convincing changes in cortical metabolism and blood flow in patients with Parkinson's disease[28]. Whether or not cortical hypometabolism is observed may well reflect the stage of the disease. In patients with early unilateral signs Wolfson et al.[29] and Perlmutter and Raichle[30] have found unilateral reductions in frontal cerebral blood flow in the hemisphere contralateral to the side with signs of parkinsonism. Wolfson et al.[29] found global reduction in cerebral blood flow in patients with bilateral signs. Striatal metabolism may be increased or normal in patients with Parkinson's disease[31].

The reductions in cortical blood flow observed in subcortical disease may well reflect reduced activation of the cortex by subcortical structures. Lesions of the thalamus[32] and caudate[33] may be associated with reductions in regional cortical cerebral metabolism or blood flow. The reductions in cerebral cortex metabolism or blood flow have been attributed to disconnection of the cortex from activating subcortical inputs. The circuitry between caudate and frontal cortex[34] may explain the effects of caudate lesions on frontal perfusion.

Neuropsychological evidence for subcortical dementia

Methodological issues

There have been several attempts to define the subcortical dementias by looking for selective cognitive impairments in these diseases using neuropsychological testing. Before discussing some of the findings in detail, the methodological issues that are pertinent to such an undertaking will be discussed.

Matching for severity of dementia Rosen[35] has commented on the problem of failing to match groups for severity of dementia. This is a major criticism of several papers that have attempted to compare the profile of neuropsychological impairments observed in patients with subcortical dementia with those with Alzheimer's disease. The populations of patients with subcortical dementia studied have tended to show mild to moderate degrees of impairment; those with Alzheimer's disease moderate to severe impairments. It should come as no surprise therefore that the Alzheimer's disease groups of patients show, statistically significant, cognitive impairments compared with control groups over a wider range of tests than do the groups with subcortical dementia.

This is illustrated by Figure 1, the hypothetical progressive cognitive impairments found in a dementia resulting from a diffuse brain disease. Tests to the right-hand side of the battery are taken to be those that are particularly vulnerable to diffuse disease. It would not be surprising if attentional tasks, possibly requiring the cooperation of widespread and distant parts of the central nervous system[36], are affected early.

With progression of this hypothetical disease, all functions will gradually become impaired, until finally there is no differential impairment across the tests, and all are performed at floor level.

Assume that all the tests show approximately the same standard deviation, and that this is the same for both control and the demented population. If one now compares the tests which are significantly different from controls for the

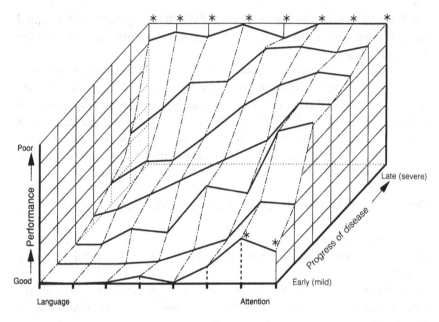

Fig. 1. Neuropsychological test battery. Asterisks indicate values significantly different from normal controls.

early mild demented groups with the late severe demented groups, then a different pattern is seen with the more severely affected populations showing impairments over a wider range of tasks. In addition, comparison of the scores of the early mild versus the late severe demented populations will also show significant differences for some tests, those only affected late in the course of the disease, but not for others. This might be interpreted as evidence that the population with early mild dementia has been afflicted with a different disease from that suffered by the population with late severe dementia. Such an interpretation would be wrong because it has not taken into account the failure to match the populations for overall severity of dementia.

This principle was nicely illustrated in two papers, looking at the same data, published by Mayeux and colleagues[37,38]. They studied the neuropsychological profile of impairments in patients with Huntington's disease and Parkinson's disease, regarded as producing subcortical dementia, and compared them with patients with Alzheimer's disease. The impairments in patients with Huntington's disease and Parkinson's disease were selective, with relative sparing of language function. This appeared to confirm the distinction between the subcortical and cortical dementias on a neuropsychological basis.

However, in the second paper they matched the three groups for overall severity. This was done because the Alzheimer's disease group showed much greater impairment overall, i.e. on the total sum score. When they did this, they could find no evidence for a differential pattern of impairment.

Huber et al.[39] have responded to the criticism that groups need to be matched for severity if meaningful analysis is to be made of differences in neuropsychological profiles of impairment, by suggesting that this would be inappropriate because one of the 'recognized' features of subcortical dementias is that they are mild[40]. Subcortical dementias may, or may not, tend to be mild. However, to show that any differences in profiles of impairment between cortical and subcortical dementias are not simply a reflection of severity of disease it is still necessary to match the groups for severity.

Ceiling effects in neuropsychological tests This methodological issue bears on the problem of matching for severity. Figure 2 is an attempt to illustrate this principle. Two tests, one easy (E) and one difficult (D), measure the same faculty (F) whose aptitude is normally distributed amongst the population. It is used to test a control population and two index populations, Mild showing mild impairments on the ability being probed by the tests, and Severe showing severe impairments. Because test E is easy it is performed at ceiling level by the control population, i.e. most subjects easily score the maximum score. The Mild group, despite being slightly impaired, also score at ceiling level. The test E therefore fails to demonstrate any differences between Mild and control populations. However, the Severe population does fall below the ceiling score and significant differences in scores between Severe and control, and Severe and Mild, are found.

The more difficult test, D, results in the control population dropping below the maximum score for that test. The slight impairment in the Mild group will now become evident because they will fail to score as efficiently as the control population. On this test Mild are significantly impaired compared with controls. The Severe group continue to be significantly impaired compared with both controls and Mild.

A different pattern of relative impairments has therefore resulted simply from the use of tests with different windows of interest. It is possible to use the same argument, but at floor levels of performance on tests, to create tests that may or may not result in Severe performing at the same level as Mild.

It is therefore important to be aware of this artefact when interpreting neuropsychological profiles of impairment across batteries of tests. Are some of the tests vulnerable to ceiling artefacts? This can only be answered if the maximum test score is known, and compared with the test scores in the study populations. If controls are achieving near maximum scores then the test is liable to ceiling effects. If the index populations being compared are not matched for overall severity then possible ceiling effects must be taken into account when comparing profiles of impairment.

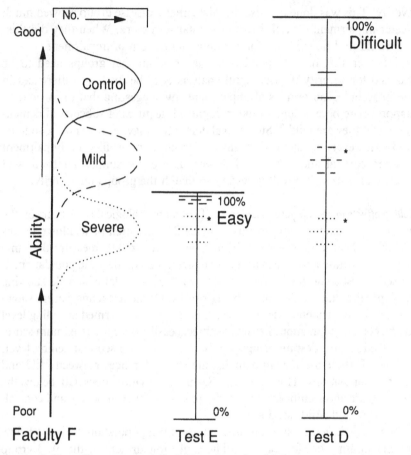

Fig. 2. Ceiling effects on psychological testing. A solid line represents the control population; a broken line represents mild impairment; a dotted line represents severe impairment. An asterisk indicates a result significantly different from controls. Means and standard errors of the means for the three groups are displayed on the lines indicating the range of possible results on the two tests, E and D.

A profile of impairments that confounds any of the methodological concerns described above is that of 'double dissociation'. This occurs when one group performs better on test A and worse on test B than does another group. Such a differential pattern of impairments cannot be explained by differences in overall severity between the two groups.

The results of Filley et al.[41] suggests a double dissociation between the impairments observed in patients with multiple sclerosis and those with Alzheimer's disease. The multiple sclerosis group had lower scores on attentional tasks, while the Alzheimer's disease group had lower scores on language tests. However, the 'scores' were not the absolute scores on the particular tests, but relative scores indicating how each subject performed on that particular test compared with their performance overall (the summed test score). On the absolute scores the Alzheimer's disease group did worse at both attentional and language tasks. The result may simply have reflected differences in severity between the groups as illustrated above.

Milberg and Albert[42] have demonstrated a valid double-dissociation between the performance of patients with Alzheimer's disease and patients with PSNP on tests evaluating naming and verbal fluency. Patients with Alzheimer's disease performed worse on tests of naming but better on tests of verbal fluency. This is good evidence of a differential pattern of neuro-psychological impairments between the two diseases.

Speed–accuracy trade off and fatigue Little attention is usually paid to these two confounding factors in the descriptions of the methodology used when administering the neuropsychological test batteries.

In many timed tests of psychomotor function the subject is faced with the choice between a slow accurate performance, or a fast performance with many errors. This may be observed in tasks that are essentially motor[43] or cogni-tive[44]. It is important to be aware of the instructions given to the patient in such tasks; whether they are instructed to perform as accurately as possible, or as quickly as possible. It is also important, when interpreting the results of such tests, to look at both the error rates and the speed of the performance. Before attributing a slow performance in one group to an impairment in function, it is necessary to ensure that group does at least as badly on error rate.

Morris et al.[44] have proposed that whether or not patients with Parkinson's disease perform slowly or inaccurately on certain cognitive tests depends on whether or not the goal of the test is implicit or explicit. On tests in which the goal is explicit, i.e. in which there are clear instructions as to what the subject is expected to do, they perform the test slowly but accurately. However, in tests with implicit goals they perform badly in their attempt to determine the rules of the test. A good example of a test with implicit goals is the Wisconsin Card Sorting test. The subject has to work out the rules for sorting the cards from the pattern of correct/incorrect responses that his initial attempts to sort the cards generates. Patients with Parkinson's disease produce more errors in their attempts to follow the, implicitly, changing rules.

The personality of the subject may also play a part in determining the test scores. Obsessional subjects will tend to perform accurately at the expense of speed. There is some evidence that patients with Parkinson's disease may be rigid and obsessional[45], and this may bias their pattern of responding in some neuropsychological tests. Possibly patients with Alzheimer's disease, showing little concern, may respond quickly, at the expense of more errors in their performance.

Readiness to fatigue will interact with the order of test presentation to affect test scores. If the tests are always presented in the same order to all subjects then one group may perform less well on the later tests simply as a result of greater fatigue. Fatigue is a common symptom in multiple sclerosis[46] and Parkinson's disease[47]. Jennekens-Schinkel et al.[48] demonstrated that the reaction time of patients with multiple sclerosis increased after 4 hours of psychological testing. Careful studies therefore vary the order of neuropsychological testing to exclude order effects[49].

Ascertainment bias Suppose a study on Alzheimer's disease recruits most of the patients in the study group from a memory clinic. It should come as no surprise to find that the population of Alzheimer's disease studied has selective memory impairments. The patients with Alzheimer's disease have come to the attention of the researcher *because* they have memory deficits! This is an example of ascertainment bias.

Studies that have demonstrated significant differences between subcortical and cortical dementias have compared the neuropsychological profile of patients with Alzheimer's disease ('cortical'), with patients with a movement disorder (e.g. Parkinson's disease) who have been found, on investigation, to show evidence of cognitive impairment ('subcortical'). The Alzheimer patients are almost invariably recruited from hospital services. The studies are therefore open to the criticism that the patients with Alzheimer's dementia that they are studying may be a selected group of Alzheimer patients, i.e. those with cognitive or behavioural problems that provoke referral to hospital services. It seems not unlikely that patients with Alzheimer's disease with disturbance of cortical functions, e.g. aphasia or agnosia, will present early to hospital services. Those who only show difficulties with concentrating or forgetfulness or slowness of mentation will be regarded as simply 'getting old' because such symptoms are common in the normal elderly[2]. They will therefore tend not to be referred to specialist services.

No such referral bias is likely to have been operating in the group of patients with 'subcortical' dementia, who have presented with a movement disorder that almost invariably results in referral to hospital. Any differences in neuropsychological profiles between the two groups, even when they are matched for overall severity, may therefore simply reflect poor performance in the Alzheimer group in subtests which, when impaired, result in early referral to hospital.

That such a referral bias has room to manoeuvre is suggested by reports that five times more elderly suffering from dementia are at home than in institutions[50].

Bergmann et al.[51] compared symptom profiles in hospital and community resident elderly patients with dementia. They found a rather different profile of impairments in the two groups. The hospital group showed more 'memory impairment', 'disorientation' and 'lack of insight'.

Further study on the differences between hospital and community based population of patients with Alzheimer's disease is needed to ensure that ascertainment bias is not accounting for the differences that are found between patients with subcortical disease and patients with Alzheimer's disease.

Neuropsychological evidence

The large neuropsychological literature on the deficits observed in the various subcortical diseases will not be fully reviewed here. Brown and Marsden[52] have reviewed in detail the evidence for the validity of the concept of subcortical dementia. They looked only at studies that have directly compared at least two groups of patients from those with Alzheimer's disease, Parkinson's disease or Huntington's disease, on neuropsychological tests. Their conclusion was that the overall similarities btween Alzheimer's disease, Parkinson's disease, and Huntington's disease tend to override their differences; and that the similarity between Huntington's disease and Parkinson's disease is not strikingly greater than the differences between these two and Alzheimer's disease.

Nevertheless there is good evidence that disorders of attention, activation and alertness, psychomotor speed, 'set-shifting', sequencing and temporal organization are prominent in diseases which damage subcortical structures in the cerebral hemispheres and brainstem. One of the goals of comparative neuropsychology is to dissect out the differences in impairments in such a way that selective dysfunction can be attributed to disturbance of particular systems in the brain, be they neuroanatomical or neurochemical.

This has resulted in research workers looking for psychological abnormalities that are specific to individual diseases. An example is the attempt to define the disturbance observed in Parkinson's disease. Deficits in temporal ordering[53], internal versus external cueing[54] or extra-dimensional, as opposed to intra-dimensional, shifting[55] have been found in Parkinson's disease. It is tempting to speculate on the relation between such observations in humans, and the relatively well defined study of dopamine systems on psychological function in animals. However, before doing so research workers should be aware of their obligation to ensuring that the dysfunction is indeed specific to Parkinson's disease. Are the findings common to all subcortical diseases, or singular to Parkinson's disease?

The comparative neuropsychology of Parkinson's disease and multiple sclerosis may be used to illustrate this principle. Patients with Parkinson's disease are often regarded as showing bradyphrenia, a slowing of thought processes, and dopamine depletion has been proposed as being of fundamen-

S Fleminger

Table 1. *Bradyphrenia in Parkinson's disease*

No	Yes
1. *Choice reaction time versus simple reaction time*	
Evarts et al.[61]	Pullman et al.[65a]
Bloxham et al.[62]	
Rafal et al.[63]	
Girotti et al.[64]	
Dubois et al.[60]	
2. *Memory scanning*[a]	
Rafal et al.[63]	Wilson et al.[65]†
3. *Trails B–A*[b]	
Heitanen & Teravainen[66]	Heitanen & Teravainen[66]‡
Taylor et al.[67]	Taylor et al.[68]§
4. *Letter cancellation*	
Horne[69]	Talland & Schwab[70]
5. *Digit symbol substitution*[c]	
	Rogers et al.[56]″
6. *Indirect evidence*	
	Sagar et al.[53]i
	Sahakian et al.[71]ii
	Morris et al.[44]iii

Notes on Table 1:
* Choice reaction time selectively improved by L-dopa.
† Found only in older group of patients.
‡ Slowing only observed in patients with disease onset less than 60 years.
§ Slowing only observed in patients with poor response to L-dopa.
″ Slowing controlled for movement time.
Indirect evidence:
  i Constant impaired performance over first 6 seconds of recall task.
  ii Delay independent impairment over first 8 seconds of delayed match to sample.
  iii Increased planning time to first move on Tower of London.
References to tests:
[a] Sternberg[72]
[b] Reitan trail making test; Halstead[73]
[c] WAIS digit symbol substitution (modified): Wechsler[74]

tal importance[56]. However, the study of mental processing speed in patients with multiple sclerosis (Table 2) has revealed a similar pattern of slowing, across various tests, to that observed in patients with Parkinson's disease (Table 1). It would appear that bradyphrenia on complex mental tasks is common to both Parkinson's disease and multiple sclerosis. Theories of bradyphrenia that are not able to accommodate these findings need to be treated with caution.

Table 2. *Bradyphrenia in multiple sclerosis*

No	Yes
1. *Choice reaction time versus simple reaction time*	
Jennekens et al.[48]	Lehman et al.[75]
van den Burg et al.[49]*	
2. *Memory scanning*[a]	
Litvan et al.[76]	Rao et al.[77]†
3. *Trails B–A*[b]	
van den Burg et al.[49]*	Grant et al.[78]
4. *Letter cancellation*	
	Medaer et al.[79]
5. *Digit symbol substitution*[c]	Beatty et al.[80]‡
6. *Indirect evidence*	
	Litvan et al.[81]i

Notes on Table 2:
* Slowing of mental speed is not present when results covaried for motor speed.
† Slowing correlates with thickness of corpus callosum.
‡ Verbal response.
Indirect evidence:
i Impaired recency effect on recall of 5 word list.
References to tests:
[a] Sternberg[72]
[b] Reitan trail making test; Halstead[73]
[c] WAIS digit symbol substitution (modified): Wechsler[74]

Conclusions

The concept of a syndrome of subcortical dementia has been of great value in promoting research which has considered the role of subcortical structures in normal mental life and cognitive function. There can be no doubt that individual differences have conspired to make an objective delineation of the syndrome difficult. Not only do individuals react to identical cerebral insults with different patterns of mental symptoms and cognitive dysfunction, but disorders that are generally regarded as producing essentially identical cerebral lesions may in fact be quite heterogenous in their pathology. This latter principle is well illustrated by the neuropathology of Parkinson's disease; there may be variable involvement of cerebral cortex or brainstem nuclei with plaques and tangles[57], or with Lewy bodies[58,59]. Another example of the heterogeneity of disease processes is the case presented by Salmon and Frank[22]. They described the PET scan findings in a patient with Pick's disease who presented with an aphasia; the scan early in the course of the disease showed selective left perisylvian hypometabolism. Only later in the course of the disease was the typical bilateral fronto-temporal hypometabol-

S Fleminger

ism of Pick's disease observed; a biopsy showed typical Pick's neuropathology (PSNP).

Albert and colleagues'[12] choice of PSNP as the disease producing the
archetypal subcortical dementia seems to have been appropriate. Of all the
diseases that produce this syndrome, the clinical picture produced by PSNP
is the most characteristic of the syndrome, and the most readily defined as
being distinct from cortical dementia. For example Dubois et al.[60] were able
to demonstrate bradyphrenia in patients with PSNP in a choice versus simple
reaction time task, while patients with Parkinson's disease failed to show
bradyphrenia on this task, as noted in Table 1. Patients with PSNP also did
worse on the Wisconsin Card Sorting test; this latter finding is compatible
with the consistent hypometabolism of frontal cortex observed in PSNP (see
above).

Patients with PSNP perform badly on tests of verbal fluency compared
with tests of naming[42]; again consistent with impairment of frontal lobe
function in PSNP. As noted above it was this study that was able to
demonstrate a double dissociation between the impairments found in PSNP
and those found in Alzheimer's disease. Again this is very good evidence that
the dementia of PSNP is different in *type* from that of Alzheimer's disease,
and not simply in *degree*. Clinical impression is that patients with PSNP are
particularly likely to show apathy and depression.

However, it now seems reasonable to abandon the debate as to whether or
not subcortical dementia exists. Studies which throw large batteries of
standard psychological tests at groups of patients with different diseases
appear to be of limited value. More valuable are those that are able to define
out a double dissociations of psychological impairments, or in which attempts
are made to develop tests to explore specific theories of brain function that can
be tested by studying patients with cerebral disease.

References

(1) Kendell RE. *The role of diagnosis in psychiatry*. Oxford: Blackwell Scientific Publications, 1975: 4.
(2) Albert MS. Subcortical dementia. In: Katzman R, Terry RD, Bick KL, eds. *Alzheimer's disease: senile dementia and related disorders*. New York: Raven Press, 1978: 173–80.
(3) Navia BA, Jordan BD, Price RW. The AIDS dementia complex. 1. Clinical features. *Ann Neurol* 1986; 19: 517–24.
(4) Rao SM. Neuropsychology of multiple sclerosis: a critical review. *J Clin Exp Neuropsychol* 1986; 8: 503–46.
(5) Junque C, Pujol J, Vendrell P, et al. Leukoaraiosis on magnetic resonance imaging and speed of mental processing. *Arch Neurol* 1990; 47: 151–6.
(6) Benson DF. Subcortical dementia: a clinical approach. In: Mayeux R, Rosen WG, eds. *The dementias*. New York: Raven Press, 1983; *Adv Neurol* 38: 185–94.
(7) Van Gorp WG, Mitrushina M, Cummings JL, Satz P, Modesitt J. Normal

ageing and the subcortical encephalopathy of AIDS. *Neuropsychiat Neuropsychol Behav Neurol* 1989; 2: 5–20.

(8) Filley CM, Franklin GM, Heaton RK, Rosenberg NL. White matter dementia: clinical disorders and implications. *Neuropsychiat Neuropsychol Behav Neurol* 1989; 1: 239–54.

(9) Gupta SR, Naheedy MH, Young JC, Ghobrial M, Rubino FA, Hindo W. Periventricular white matter changes and dementia. Clinical, neuropsychological, radiological and pathological correlation. *Arch Neurol* 1988; 45: 637–41.

(10) Mader JT. Neurobehavioural and magnetic resonance imaging findings in two cases of decompression sickness. *Aviat Space Environ Med* 1989; 60: 1204–10.

(11) Cummings JL, Benson DF. Psychological dysfunction accompanying Subcortical dementia. *Ann Rev Med* 1988; 39: 53–61.

(12) Albert ML, Feldman RG, Willis AL. The subcortical dementia of progressive supranuclear palsy. *J Neurol Neurosurg Psychiat* 1974; 37: 121–30.

(13) Laplane D, Baulac M, Widlocher D, Dubois B. Pure psychic akinesia with bilateral lesions of the basal ganglia. *J Neurol Neurosurg Psychiat* 1984; 47: 377–85.

(14) Richfield EK, Twyman R, Berent S. Neurological syndrome following bilateral damage to head of the caudate nuclei. *Ann Neurol* 1987; 22: 718.

(15) Strub RL. Frontal lobe syndrome in a patient with bilateral *Globus pallidus* lesions. *Arch Neurol* 1989; 46: 1024–7.

(16) Lishman WA. *Organic psychiatry: the psychological consequences of cerebral disorder. 2nd ed.* Oxford: Blackwell Scientific Publications, 1987.

(17) Reifler BV, Larson E, Hanley R. Coexistence of cognitive impairment and depression in geriatric outpatients. *Am J Psychiat* 1982; 139: 623–6.

(18) Lazarus LW, Newton N, Cohler B, Lesser J, Schweon C. Frequency and presentation of depressive symptoms in patients with primary degenerative dementia. *Am J Psychiat* 1987; 144: 41–5.

(19) Striano S, Meo R, Bilo L. Conventional EEG in the differential diagnosis of dementia syndromes. *Acta Neurol (Napoli)* 1988; 10: 98–107.

(20) Flowers CJ, Harrison MJG. EEG changes in subcortical dementia: a study of 22 patients with Steele–Richardson–Olszewski (SRO) syndrome. *Electroenceph Cl Neurophysiol* 1986; 64: 301–3.

(21) Goodin DS, Aminoff MJ. The distinction between different types of dementia using evoked potentials. *Electroenceph Cl Neurophysiol* 1987; *(Suppl)* 40; 695–8.

(22) Salmon E, Frank G. Positron emission tomography in degenerative dementias. *Acta Neurol Belg* 1989; 89: 150–5.

(23) Kuhl DE, Phelps ME, Markham CH, Metter EJ, Riege WH, Winter J. Cerebral metabolism and atrophy in Huntington's disease determined by 18FDG and computed tomographic scans. *Ann Neurol* 1982; 12: 425–34.

(24) Weinberger DR, Berman KF, Iadarola MA, Driesen N, Zec RF. Prefrontal cortical blood flow and cognitive function in Huntington's disease. *J Neurol Neurosurg Psychiat* 1988; 51: 94–104.

(25) D'Antona R, Baron JC, Samson Y, et al. Subcortical dementia: frontal cortex hypometabolism detected by positron emission tomography in patients with progressive supranuclear palsy. *Brain* 1985; 108: 785–9.

(26) Leenders KL, Frackowiak RSJ, Lees AJ. Steele–Richardson–Olszewski syn-

drome: Brain energy metabolism, blood flow and fluorodopa uptake measured by positron emission tomography. *Brain* 1988; 111: 615–30.

(27) Goffinet AM, De Volder AG, Gillain C, Rectem D, Bol A, Michel C, Cogneau M, Labar D, Laterre C. Positron tomography demonstrates frontal lobe hypometabolism in Progressive Supranuclear palsy. *Ann Neurol* 1989; 25: 131–9.

(28) Martin WRW, Stoessl AJ, Adam MJ, et al. Positron emission tomography in Parkinson's disease: glucose and DOPA metabolism. *Adv Neurol* 1986; 45: 95–8.

(29) Wolfson LI, Leenders KL, Brown LL, Jones T. Alterations of regional cerebral blood flow and oxygen metabolism in Parkinson's disease. *Neurology* 1985; 35: 1399–405.

(30) Perlmutter JS, Raichle ME. Regional blood flow in hemiparkinsonism. *Neurology* 1985; 35: 1127–34.

(31) Brooks DJ, Frackowiak RSJ. PET and movement disorders. *J Neurol Neurosurg Psychiat* 1989 (June suppl.): 68–77.

(32) D'Antona R, Baron JC, Pantano P, Serdaru M, Bousser MG, Samson Y. Effects of thalamic lesions on cerebral cortex metabolism in humans. *J Cereb Blood Flow Metab* 1985; 5 (Suppl. 1): s457–8.

(33) Pozilli C, Passafiume D, Bastianello S, D'Antona R, Lenzi GL. Remote effects of caudate haemorrhage: a clinical and functional study. *Cortex* 1987; 23: 341–9.

(34) Alexander GE, DeLong MR, Strick PL. Parallel organisation of functionally segregated circuits linking basal ganglia and cortex. *Ann Rev Neuroscience* 1986; 9: 357–81.

(35) Rosen TJ. Cortical versus subcortical dementia: neuropsychological similarities. *Arch Neurol* 1987; 44: 131.

(36) Mesulam M-M. A cortical network for directed attention and unilateral neglect. *Ann Neurol* 1981; 10: 309–25.

(37) Mayeux R, Stern Y, Rosen J, Benson DF. Subcortical dementia: a recognizable clinical entity. *Ann Neurol* 1981; 10: 100–1A.

(38) Mayeux R, Stern Y, Rosen J, Benson DF. Is 'subcortical dementia' a recognizable clinical entity. *Ann Neurol* 1983; 14: 278–83.

(39) Huber SJ, Shuttleworth EC, Paulson GW. Subcortical dementia. *Arch Neurol* 1987; 44: 130.

(40) Cummings JL, Benson DF. Subcortical dementia. Review of an emerging concept. *Arch Neurol* 1984; 41: 874–9.

(41) Filley CM, Heaton RK, Nelson LM, Burks JS, Franklin GM. A comparison of dementia in Alzheimer's disease and multiple sclerosis. *Arch Neurol* 1989; 46: 157–61.

(42) Milberg W, Albert M. Cognitive differences between patients with progressive supranuclear palsy and Alzheimer's disease. *J Clin Exp Neuropsychol* 1989; 11: 605–14.

(43) Berardelli A, Accornero N, Argenta M, Meco G, Manfredi M. Fast complex arm movements in Parkinson's disease. *J Neurol Neurosurg Psychiat* 1986; 49: 1146–9.

(44) Morris RG, Downes JJ, Sahakian BJ, Evenden JL, Heald A, Robbins TW Planning and spatial working memory in Parkinson's disease. *J Neurol Neurosurg Psychiat* 1988; 51: 757–66.

(45) Todes CJ, Lees AJ. The pre-morbid personality of patients with Parkinson's disease. *J Neurol Neurosurg Psychiat* 1985; 48: 97–100.

(46) Krupp LB, Alvarez LA, LaRocca NG, Scheinberg LC. Fatigue in multiple sclerosis. *Arch Neurol* 1988; 45: 435–7.

(47) Schwab RS, England AC, Peterson E. Akinesia in Parkinson's disease. *Neurology* 1959; 9: 65–72.

(48) Jennekens-Schinkel A, Sanders EACM, Lanser JBK, Van der Velde EA. Reaction time in ambulant multiple sclerosis: Part 1 Influence of prolonged cognitive effort. *J Neurol Sci* 1988; 85: 173–86.

(49) Van den Burg W, Van Zommeren AH, Minderhoud JM, Prange AJA, Meijer NSA. Cognitive impairment in patients with multiple sclerosis and mild physical disability. *Arch Neurol* 1987; 44: 494–501.

(50) Kay DWK, Beamish P, Roth M. Old age mental disorders in Newcastle upon Tyne. Pt. 1: a study of prevalence. *Br J Psychiat* 1964; 110: 146–58.

(51) Bergmann K, Proctor S, Prudham D. Symptom profiles in hospital and community resident elderly persons with dementia. In: *Brain function in old age*. *Bayer Symposium VII*: Springer-Verlag, 1979.

(52) Brown RG, Marsden CD. 'Subcortical dementia': The neuropsychological evidence. *Neuroscience* 1988; 363–87.

(53) Sagar HJ, Sullivan EV, Gabrieli JDE, Corkin S, Growdon JH. Temporal ordering and short term memory deficits in Parkinson's disease. *Brain* 1988; 111: 525–39.

(54) Brown RG, Marsden CD. Internal versus external cues and the control of attention in Parkinson's disease. *Brain* 1988; 111: 323–30.

(55) Downes JJ, Roberts AC, Sahakian BJ, Evenden JL, Morris RG, Robbins TW. Impaired extra-dimensional shift performance in medicated and unmedicated Parkinson's disease: Evidence for a specific attentional dysfunction. *Neuropsychologia* 1989; 27: 1329–43.

(56) Rogers D, Lees AJ, Smith E, Trimble MR, Stern GM. Bradyphrenia in Parkinson's disease and psychomotor retardation in depressive illness: an experimental study. *Brain* 1987; 110: 761–76.

(57) Chui HC, Mortimer JA, Slager U, Zarow C, Bondareff W, Webster DD. Pathologic correlates of dementia in Parkinson's disease. *Arch Neurol* 1986; 43: 991–5.

(58) Jellinger K, Grisold W. Cerebral atrophy and Parkinson syndrome. *Exp Brain Res* 1982; Suppl. 5: 26–35.

(59) Gibb WRG, Esiri MM, Lees AJ. Clinical and pathological features of diffuse cortical body disease (Lewy Body Dementia). *Brain* 1987; 110: 1131–53.

(60) Dubois B, Pillon B, Legault F, Agid Y, Lhermitte F. Slowing of cognitive processing in progressive supranuclear palsy: a comparison with Parkinson's disease. *Arch Neurol* 1988; 45: 1194–9.

(61) Evarts EV, Teravainen H, Calne DB. Reaction time in Parkinson's disease. *Brain* 1981; 104: 167–86.

(62) Bloxham CA, Mindel TA, Frith CD. Initiation and execution of predictable and unpredictable movements in Parkinson's disease. *Brain* 1984; 107: 371–84.

(63) Rafal RD, Posner MI, Walker JA, Friedrich FJ. Cognition and the basal ganglia: separating mental and motor components of performance in Parkinson's disease. *Brain* 1984; 107: 1083–94.

(64) Girotti F, Carella F, Grassi MP, Soliveri P, Marano R, Caraceni T. Motor and cognitive performances of Parkinsonian patients in the on and off phases of the disease. *J Neurol Neurosurg Psychiat* 1986; 49: 657–60.

(65) Wilson RS, Kaszniak AW, Klawans HL, Garron DG. High speed memory scanning in Parkinsonism. *Cortex* 1980; 16: 67–72.

(65a) Pullman SL, Watts RL, Juncos JL, Chase TN, Sanes JN. Dopaminergic effects on simple and choice reaction time performance in Parkinson's disease. *Neurology* 1988; 38: 249–54.

(66) Heitanen M, Teravainen H. The effect of age of disease onset on neuropsychological performance in Parkinson's disease. *J Neurol Neurosurg Psychiat* 1988; 51: 244–9.

(67) Taylor AE, Saint-Cyr JA, Lang AE. Frontal lobe dysfunction in Parkinson's disease: the cortical focus of neostriatal outflow. *Brain* 1986; 109: 845–83.

(68) Taylor AE, Saint-Cyr JA, Lang AE. Parkinson's disease: Cognitive changes in relation to treatment response. *Brain* 1987; 110: 35–51.

(69) Horne DJ de L. Performance on delayed response task by patients with Parkinsonism. *J Neurol Neurosurg Psychiat* 1971; 34: 192–4.

(70) Talland GA, Schwab RS. Performance with multiple sets in Parkinson's disease. *Neuropsychologia* 1964; 2: 45–53.

(71) Sahakian BJ, Morris RG, Evenden JL, et al. A comparative study of visuospatial memory and learning in Alzheimer-type dementia and Parkinson's disease. *Brain* 1988; 111: 695–718.

(72) Sternberg S. Memory scanning: new findings and current controversies. *Quart J Exp Psychol* 1975; 27: 1–32.

(73) Halstead WC. *Brain and intelligence: a quantitative study of the frontal lobes.* Chicago: University of Chicago Press, 1947.

(74) Wechsler D. *The Wechsler adult intelligence scale (manual).* Psychological Corporation, 1955.

(75) Lehmann HJ, Glockner RJ. Cerebral disconnection in multiple sclerosis. *Eur Neurol* 1972; 8: 257–69.

(76) Litvan I, Grafman J, Vendrell P, Martinez JM. Slowed information processing in multiple sclerosis. *Arch Neurol* 1988; 45: 281–5.

(77) Rao SM, Leo GJ, Haughton VM, St Aubin-Faubert P, Bernardin L. Correlation of magnetic resonance imaging with neuropsychological testing in multiple sclerosis. *Neurology* 1989; 39: 161–6.

(78) Grant I, McDonald WI, Trimble MR, Smith E, Reed R. Deficient learning and memory in early and middle phases of multiple sclerosis. *J Neurol Neurosurg Psychiat* 1984; 47: 250–5.

(79) Medaer R, Nelivssen E, Appel B, Swerts M, Geutjen J, Callaert H. Magnetic resonance imaging and cognitive function in multiple sclerosis. *J Neurol* 1988; 235: 86–9.

(80) Beatty WW, Goodkin DE, Monson N, Beatty PA, Hertsgaard D. Anterograde and retrograde amnesia in patients with chronic progressive multiple sclerosis. *Arch Neurol* 1988; 45: 611–19.

(81) Litvan I, Grafman J, Vendrell P, et al. Multiple memory deficits in patients with multiple sclerosis: Exploring the working memory system. *Arch Neurol* 1988; 45: 607–10.

Molecular and cell biology of epilepsy

B S MELDRUM AND A G CHAPMAN

Introduction

Epilepsy appears in diverse forms associated with extremely varied primary pathologies, ranging from vascular or neuronal developmental defects to minimal or gross degenerative changes[1,2]. In the most diverse pathologies there may nevertheless be some convergence of cellular biology, not just in terms of the excessively synchronous discharge of an aggregate of neurons but also in terms of common changes of a reactive kind (e.g. selective changes in receptors, interneurons, or regenerating axons). Therapeutic response defines some cellularly different forms of epilepsy. Absence epilepsy, with 3 Hz spike and wave, is pharmacologically different from other forms of primary generalized epilepsy or focal epilepsy – its molecular and cellular basis must therefore be different and yet there is some genetic overlap with other forms of epilepsy (as in juvenile myoclonic epilepsy) and, developmentally, it may evolve into other forms of epilepsy.

Genetic basis of epilepsy

This can be considered in terms of three clinical groups. Some syndromes of primary epilepsy (i.e. in which epilepsy presents in isolation, not associated with some other developmental or acquired disorder) have a clear genetic basis. All the conditions listed in Table 1 show a rather precise developmental onset. Thus benign neonatal familial convulsions begin within the first week of life, absence attacks begin between the ages of 3 and 13 years and juvenile myoclonic epilepsies begin within the teen years. Febrile convulsions are not included in the table but also show a strong genetic predisposition, presumed to be polygenic, and a restricted age of occurrence (0.5–4.5 years). It can be said that the penetrance of the genes is age and sex dependent. (Absence epilepsy shows a higher incidence in girls than boys.) However, what is

All correspondence to: Dr BS Meldrum, Institute of Psychiatry, De Crespigny Park, Denmark Hill, London SE5 8AF, UK.

Cambridge Medical Reviews: Neurobiology and Psychiatry Volume 1
© Cambridge University Press

B S Meldrum & A G Chapman

Table 1. *Genetically determined syndromes with primary epilepsy*

Syndrome	Genetic nature	Gene location
Benign familial neonatal convulsions	Single gene Autosomal dominant	Chr 20, long arm
Benign myoclonic epilepsy in infancy	Autosomal recessive	
Absence (3 Hz sp. and wave) epilepsy	? Polygenic Autosomal dominant	
Juvenile myoclonic epilepsy	? Polygenic Autosomal dominant	Chr 6, short arm

required is a molecular explanation that can be related to developmental processes. Such an explanation may be facilitated by genetic mapping. To date, pedigree studies with genetic markers have provided evidence for the location of the gene for benign familial neonatal convulsions on chromosome 20[3] and the gene or genes for juvenile myoclonic epilepsy on chromosome 6[4]. The specific gene defect has, however, not yet been identified in either of these disorders. Possibilities would include genes coding ionic conductance channels, receptor molecules, enzymes involved in neurotransmitter metabolism or other enzymes concerned with neuronal metabolism, or genes regulating developmental processes. Some of these possibilities are discussed in more detail below.

The second clinical group are the genetically determined syndromes in which epilepsy occurs as a secondary feature with a varying incidence. These include, for example, the neurodermatoses and some other generalized or brain specific developmental disorders, and a large number of inborn errors of metabolism[2,5]. The metabolic disorders include pyridoxine dependency which responds to high doses of pyridoxine and in which the seizures are thought to result from deficient synthesis of the inhibitory transmitter (GABA) and multiple carboxylase deficiency (that responds to biotin). In these two syndromes, the link between the primary metabolic defect and the occurrence of seizures is relatively straightforward. In the various dysplastic disorders, however, the link between the primary developmental defect and the occurrence of seizures may be similar to that involved in a wide variety of secondary epilepsies (disorders of neuronal migration are discussed as a separate entity below).

The third clinical group are the primary and secondary epilepsies in which pedigree studies show an inherited element that remains largely undefined.

156

Disorders of neuronal migration

These are a particularly interesting group of disorders with 'secondary' epilepsy, partly because – unlike most disorders with secondary epilepsy – the incidence of epilepsy approaches 100% in some syndromes, and also because minor disorders of neuronal migration may be a predisposing factor in several forms of epilepsy. Disorders of neuronal migration most commonly have a genetic cause but intrauterine factors are also significant (including viral infections such as cytomegalovirus (CMV)). Migration of neurons through the cortex occurs during the third, fourth and fifth months of gestation, and involves several biochemical systems, including the cell adhesion molecules. Defects can be classified into broad morphological types. Lissencephaly (agyria/pachygyria) has been divided into two types[6,7], Type I lissencephaly has a cortex of four layers: heterotopic non-migrated neurons, a cell-sparse layer, a layer corresponding to laminae III, V and VI and an outer, molecular layer. When combined with specific facial and somatic dysmorphisms this is known as Miller–Dieker syndrome and is associated with a mini-deletion on the short arm of chromosome 17 (partial monosomy 17, p13). Lissencephaly type II shows almost complete absence of cortical lamination and falls into several subtypes according to the associated malformations (hydrocephalus, retinal dysplasia, muscle disorders) which are autosomal recessive disorders. Type I lissencephaly is associated with a very high incidence of epilepsy; seizures and infantile spasms usually start in the first 6 months of life in the Miller–Dieker syndrome.

Tuberous sclerosis is associated with a very high incidence of epilepsy, indeed seizures or infantile spasms are the commonest presenting syndrome. It is an autosomal dominant condition; linkage analysis has identified two gene loci, both of which are near the genes for adhesion molecules (locus 11q23 near the gene for NCAM and locus 9q34 near the gene for tenacin)[8]. This might explain the observed defective neuronal migration with heterotopia.

The minimal disorder of neuronal migration is a neuronal heterotopia with clusters of neurons in the subcortical white matter.

A very minor degree of this is probably normal but a greater degree can be identified in operative or post-mortem material from patients with several forms of epilepsy. Thus marked heterotopia was found by Hardiman et al in 42% of temporal lobectomy specimens from patients with intractable temporal lobe epilepsy (and in none of 33 neurologically normal autopsy brains)[9]. It would thus appear to be a possible predisposing factor to temporal lobe epilepsy. Even more striking is the high incidence of 'microdysgenesis' (which includes large 'dystopic' neurons in superficial laminae, architectural disturbances in superficial and deep laminae as well as subcortical heterotopia) described by Meenke in primary generalized epilepsy (11 out of 12 children with absence epilepsy, 2 out of 3 with juvenile myoclonic epilepsy)[10]. The microdysgenesis can be presumed to be genetically determined and may be the link responsible for epileptogenesis.

Mesial temporal sclerosis

Hippocampal or mesial temporal sclerosis is the most characteristic pathological finding in the brains of patients with epilepsy dying in institutions (Margerison & Corsellis, 1966)[11] and in anterior temporal lobectomy specimens removed for intractable complex partial seizures[12]. It is characterized by a selective loss of pyramidal neurons in the CA1 and CA3–4 subfields of the hippocampus, and sometimes by neuronal loss and gliosis in some amygdala nuclei. Removal of tissue containing this pathology commonly leads to disappearance of the seizures. It appears highly probable that the lesion plays an important role in the causation of intractable temporal lobe seizures. Controversy, however, surrounds both the mechanism responsible for inducing the lesion and the mechanism by which the lesion causes seizures. In rodents and experimental primates hippocampal sclerosis can be induced by prolonged seizures either generalized or confined to the limbic system (induced by a wide range of convulsants including allylglycine, bicuculline, pilocarpine and kainate). The cell loss appears to be a direct consequence of the excessive neuronal activity associated with the local epileptic activity[13] through an excitotoxic mechanism[14]. Prolonged convulsions in infancy or childhood appear to be the most probable cause of the hippocampal sclerosis found in patients with temporal lobe epilepsy. Febrile convulsions are particularly significant if prolonged and asymetric, but non-febrile convulsions may also be important. A history of febrile convulsions, usually prolonged, is obtained in more than 50% of patients that show hippocampal sclerosis as the primary lesion at temporal lobectomy[12,15–18]. In one study[19] the cell loss was assessed quantitatively for the hippocampal subfields in 32 lobectomy specimens and correlated with clinical history. In 13 of the 32 specimens there was severe cell loss in CA1, in the endfolium and in the dentate gyrus, all 13 were associated with a severe first seizure in the first two years of life.

Conversely, magnetic resonance imaging in patients with temporal lobe epilepsy giving a history of a prolonged febrile convulsion (between the ages of 3 months and five years) consistently reveals unilateral hippocampal sclerosis[20].

If it is true that the hippocampal cell loss associated with temporal lobe epilepsy occurs in early childhood (or even in the perinatal period, as some believe) why do the complex partial seizures start only in later childhood? It certainly appears that the cell loss itself is not directly responsible for the seizures, but may induce secondary processes that in time favour focal epileptogenesis. These possibilities include regenerative changes (such as 'sprouting' of axons) and changes in membranes and receptor mechanisms.

Sprouting

This process has been studied in most detail in the hippocampus, particularly the mossy fibre system that is comprised of the axons of dentate granule cells. It occurs following cell loss in CA3 (the principal target area for the granule cell axons) induced by the focal or intracerebro-ventricular injection of kainate[21]. It can also be induced by electrical kindling of seizures by stimulation of the amygdala or perforant path, a process which leads to cell loss in the endfolium[22,23]. In temporal lobectomy specimens sprouting of the mossy fibre system has been studied by Timm's staining for zinc (which is found in high concentration in the mossy fibre system) or by dynorphin immunochemistry[24,25]. Both methods reveal a dense new innervation of the inner third of the dentate molecular layer and of the CA1 dendritic fields. Although it has been suggested that such sprouting provides a recurrent excitatory input to the dentate granule cells, there is both morphological and physiological evidence that the endings activate basket cells which are inhibitory. Thus its role in the causation of intractable seizures remains uncertain.

Immunocytochemical studies reveal a selective loss of certain categories of hilar interneuron (those containing somatostatin and neuropeptide Y) in human temporal lobe epilepsy[26]. It has been suggested[27,28] that these neurons are part of an inhibitory feed back loop within the hilus of the hippocampus and that their impairment can lead to a failure of inhibitory function, in the presence of normal GABAergic neurons (see below).

GABAergic deficits

A primary function of the recurrent inhibitory system provided by intrinsic GABAergic neurons in the cortex and hippocampus is the prevention of the excessively sustained or synchronous discharge of the principal neurons. Evidence for this is provided by the powerful epileptogenic effect of drugs that block the synthesis or postsynaptic action of GABA, and the anticonvulsant action of agents enhancing GABAergic function, such as the anticonvulsant benzodiazepines and β-carbolines. Thus defects in GABAergic systems are potential primary causes of epilepsy. Among genetic syndromes pyridoxine dependent convulsions have already received mention. Now that the GABA/benzodiazepine receptor has been cloned and sequenced[29] it has become apparent that the receptor complex is heteromeric and that the different subunits exist in many genetically distinct forms. Thus there is the possibility for a range of mild to severe genetically determined changes in the properties of the GABA-benzodiazepine receptor. Such genetic abnormalities have not yet been identified in man. There are many genetic syndromes manifesting seizures in rodents. Some abnormalities in the GABA/benzodiazepine receptors have been detected by autoradiographic means, e.g. in DBA/2 mice and in gerbils[30,31]. These syndromes appear, however, to manifest abnormalities in several transmitter systems. It is unlikely that the primary genetic defect is in a gene coding for the GABA/benzodiazepine receptor.

An acquired deficit in the GABAergic system has frequently been proposed as a cause of epilepsy[32]. The clearest anatomical evidence for such a deficit concerns focal epilepsy induced by cortical application of alumina in the monkey. Immunocytochemical labelling of glutamic acid decarboxylase positive cell bodies or puncta (terminals) shows a loss of GABAergic neurons and terminals in and around the focus[33,33a]. Although doubts have been expressed about the selectivity of such damage, it has been shown to commence prior to the onset of focal seizure discharges[34].

In material resected from human cortex or hippocampus recent studies indicate a relative preservation of GABAergic neurons[35] rather than a selective loss, as proposed earlier on the basis of biochemical measurements[32].

Abnormalities in excitatory neurotransmission

There are many ways in which enhanced excitatory activity might contribute to epileptic phenomena. The paroxysmal depolarizing shift that underlies burst firing in epileptic foci[36] has many of the characteristics of a giant excitatory post-synaptic potential. It is closely mimicked by the ionophoretic application of n-methyl-d-aspartate (NMDA) to neurons in the hippocampus, cortex or striatum[37]. Thus enhanced sensitivity of the NMDA receptor system could be an important factor in epileptogenesis. Indirect evidence that the NMDA receptor may play a role in epileptogenesis is provided by the potent anti-epileptic action of NMDA receptor antagonists[38,39]. More direct evidence in support of this hypothesis comes from autoradiographic and electrophysiological observations in human material. Temporal lobectomy specimens have been used to study the density and distribution of the sub-types of glutamate receptor (in comparison to autopsy controls). One study found a relative loss of kainate and NMDA receptors in the sclerotic regions (hilus, CA3 and CA1) presumably a direct result of cell loss, but an increase in the density of kainate and NMDA receptors in the parahippocampal gyrus[40]. Another study, presumably with less severely lesioned hippocampi, found that NMDA receptors were enhanced in density (as judged both from [³H]-glutamate binding and strychnine-insensitive [³H]-glycine binding), is increased in area CA1 and the dentate gyrus of hippocampi from temporal lobe epilepsy patients[41]. These studies suggest that there may be some kind of upregulation of NMDA receptors in patients with intractable temporal lobe epilepsy. They do not, however, provide information about the functional state of the receptors. In vitro electrophysiological studies using cortical slices from patients with or without focal epilepsy have however provided evidence for functional changes in the NMDA receptor system. The method used by Louvel and Pumain[42] employs ion-sensitive electrodes to measure the extra-cellular concentration of calcium $[Ca^{2+}]_o$. This decreases as a result of activation of NMDA receptors. Iontophoresis of NMDA at different depths in the cortex provides a functional chart of the effect of activation of the NMDA receptors. Normally, the effect is maximal in the superficial laminae but in cortex from epileptic foci enhanced sensitivity to NMDA is seen in the deeper cortical laminae.

Studies of hippocampal slices from kindled rats also indicate an increased sensitivity to NMDA either in the dentate granule cells[43] or in the CA3 pyramidal neurons[44]. This is clearly one of a number of acquired abnormalities in synaptic function in the kindled hippocampus. Although it is probably not a unique determinant of the kindled state it may nevertheless be an important contributory factor.

Membrane conductance abnormalities

There has been a remarkable increase in recent years in the number of membrane conductances that can be separately identified. In particular a range of conductances for Na^+, K^+ and Ca^{2+} may be involved in epileptogenesis. Abnormalities in such conductance mechanisms could be genetically determined or could be the secondary consequence of other metabolic abnormalities. The low-threshold Ca^{2+} conductance contributes importantly to rhythmic firing in thalamic neurons[45]. It is probably involved in 3 Hz spike and wave discharges. The transient low-threshold calcium current is reduced by drugs specifically therapeutic in absence seizures (such as the succinimides)[46]. The therapeutic action of ethosuximide is thought to be due to reduction of this calcium current; whether an abnormality in this conductance underlies absence seizures is not however, known.

Recombinant breeding experiments in DBA/2 mice have suggested that the seizure susceptibility is closely linked to a genetic abnormality influencing expression of calcium-ATPase activity[47].

Network abnormalities and consequences of activity

In the very complex networks of inhibitory and excitatory pathways of the cortex or hippocampus the final outcome of a synchronous pattern of firing of output neurons could arise in many different ways. Among these are changes in the neuronal membrane properties, for example voltage or ion sensitivities of particular conductance channels, changes in inhibitory or excitatory synaptic function, and changes in the connectivity of the network. Any of these types of change could arise as a consequence of particular patterns of activity, for example by producing changes in ionic concentrations or by producing desensitization or habituation of particular systems. Also many receptors and conductance channels have their properties altered by phosphorylation, and various protein kinases are activated following enhanced neuronal activity. There is also an effect of activity on gene expression. This is particularly clearly seen in terms of immediate early genes directly after seizure activity. Thus the c-*fos* and *jun* genes are turned on in dentate granule cells by hippo-campal epileptic activity, probably through enhanced Ca^{2+} entry to the nucleus and kinase activation. This effect can be seen 30 min after a pentylenetetrazol-induced seizure, but a 30 s afterdischarge is sufficient to produce induction of the c-*fos* gene[48].

The immediate early genes act to induce various target genes, including the genes for preproenkephalin and preprodynorphin, and for trophic factors such as NGF[49]. Thus transiently enhanced activity, particularly after discharges or brief seizures can give rise to more enduring changes in the synthesis of peptide neurotransmitters or of trophic factors which in turn will modify the properties of the neuronal network.

Conclusion: Cellular and molecular basis of epilepsy

Although we cannot give precise molecular explanations for most syndromes of epilepsy, we can offer a wide variety of partial or tentative explanations. These concern, among others, ionic conductance mechanisms, receptor complexes for inhibitory and excitatory neurotransmission, protein kinases or phosphatases and other enzymes modifying ionophore or receptor function. Abnormalities in these systems could arise directly through the expression of an abnormal gene or indirectly through a variety of mechanisms. Approaches employing the techniques of molecular biology to genetically determined forms of epilepsy (both in man and other animals) are likely to identify specific abnormal genes that may be shown to code for some of the molecules discussed or may involve entirely unsuspected mechanisms.

References

(1) Dreifuss FE, Martinez-Lage M, Roger J, Seino M, Wolf P, Dam M. Proposal for classification of epilepsies and epileptic syndromes. *Epilepsia* 1985; 26: 268–78.

(2) Engel J. *Seizures and epilepsy* FA Davis Company, 1989: Philadelphia. 1–536.

(3) Leppert M, Anderson VE, Quattlebaum T, et al. Benign familial neonatal convulsions linked to genetic markers on chromosome 20. *Nature* 1989; 337: 647–8.

(4) Delgado-Escueta AV, Greenberg D, Weissbecker K, et al. Gene mapping in the idiopathic generalised epilepsies: juvenile myoclonic epilepsy, childhood absence epilepsy, epilepsy with grand mal seizures, and early childhood myoclonic epilepsy. *Epilepsia* 1990; 31 (suppl 3): S19–S29.

(5) McKusick E. *Mendelian inheritance in man.* London: Heinemann Medical, 1983.

(6) Barth PG. Disorders of neuronal migration. *Can J Neurol Sci* 1987; 14: 1–16.

(7) Dobyns WB, Stratton RF, Greenberg F. Syndromes with lissencephaly I. Miller-Dieker and Norma-Roberts syndrome and isolated lissencephaly. *Am J Med Genet* 1984; 18: 509–26.

(8) Editorial. Progress in tuberous sclerosis. *Lancet* 1990; 336: 598–9.

(9) Hardiman O, Burke T, Phillips J, et al. Microdysgenesis in resected temporal cortex: incidence and clinical significance in focal epilepsy. *Neurology* 1988; 38: 1041–7.

(10) Meenke HJ. Pathology of childhood epilepsies. *Clev Clin J Med* 1990; 56 (suppl 1): S111–S20.

(11) Margerison JH, Corsellis JAN. Epilepsy and the temporal lobes. *Brain* 1966; 89: 499–530.

(12) Bruton CJ. *The neuropathology of temporal lobe epilepsy*, New York: Oxford University Press, 1968.

(13) Meldrum BS. Cell damage in epilepsy and the role of calcium in cytotoxicity. In: Delgado-Escueta AV, Ward AA, Jr, Woodbury DM, Porter RJ, eds. *Advances in neurology*, New York: Raven Press, 1986; 849–55.

(14) Meldrum BS, Garthwaite J. Excitatory amino acid neurotoxicity and neurode-generative disease. *TIPS* 1990; 11: 379–87.

(15) Falconer MA. Mesial temporal (Ammon's horn) sclerosis as a common cause of epilepsy. Aetiology, treatment and prevention. *Lancet* 1974; 11: 767–70.

(16) Duncan JS, Sagar HJ. Seizure characteristics, pathology, and outcome after temporal lobectomy. *Neurology* 1987; 37: 405–9.

(17) Kim JH, Guimaraes, PO, Shen MY, Masukawa LM, and Spencer DD. Hippo-campal neuronal density in temporal lobe epilepsy with and without gliomas. *Acta Neuropath.* (Berl) 1990; 80: 41–5.

(18) Ounsted C, Lindsay J, Norman R. *Biological factors in temporal lobe epilepsy*, London: Heinemann Medical Books Ltd, 1966.

(19) Sagar HJ, Oxbury JM. Hippocampal neuron loss in temporal lobe epilepsy: correlation with early childhood convulsions. *Ann Neurol* 1987; 22: 334–40.

(20) Berkovic SF, Andermann F, Olivier, et al. Hippocampal sclerosis in temporal lobe epilepsy demonstrated by magnetic resonance imaging. *Ann Neurol* 1991; 29: 175–82.

(21) Nadler JV, Martin D, Bowe MA, Marrisett RA, McNamara JO. Kindling, prenatal exposure to alcohol and postnatal development selectively alter responses of hippocampal pyramidal cells to NMDA. In: Ben-Ari Y, ed. *Excitatory amino acids and neuronal plasticity*, New York: Plenum Press, 1990: 1–10.

(22) Sutula T, He XX, Cavazos J, Scott G. Synaptic reorganisation induced in the hippocampus by abnormal functional activity. *Science* 1988; 239: 1147–50.

(23) Cavazos JE, Sutla TP. Progressive neuronal loss induced by kindling: a possible mechanism for mossy fiber synaptic reorganisation and hippocampal sclerosis. *Brain Res* 1990; 527: 1–6.

(24) Sutual T, Cascino G, Cavazos J, Parada I, Ramirez L. Mossy fiber synaptic reorganisation in the epileptic human temporal lobe. *Ann Neurol* 1989; 26: 321–30.

(25) Houser CR, Miyzshiro JE, Swartz BE, Walsh GO, Rich JR, Delgado-Escueta AV. Altered patterns of dynorphin immunoreactivity suggest mossy fiber reorganisation in human hippocampal epilepsy. *J Neurosci* 1990; 10: 267–82.

(26) DeLanerolle NC, Kim JH, Robbins RJ, Spencer DD. Hippocampal inter-neuron loss and plasticity in human temporal lobe epilepsy. *Brain Res* 1989; 495: 387–95.

B S Meldrum & A G Chapman

(27) Sloviter RS. Chemically defined hippocampal interneurons and their possible relationship to seizure mechanisms. In: Chan-Palay V, Kohler C, eds. *The hippocampus – new vistas*, Alan R Liss, 1989: 443–61.

(28) Sloviter RS. Feedforward and feedback inhibition of hippocampal principal cell activity evoked by perforant path stimulation; GABA-mediated mechanisms that regulate excitability in vivo. Hippocampus 1991; 1:31–40.

(29) Schofield PR, Darlison MG, Fujita N, et al. Sequence and functional expression of the GABA A receptor shows a ligand-gated receptor super-family. *Nature* 1987; 328: 221–7.

(30) Horton RW, Prestwich SA, Meldrum BS. γ Aminobutyric acid and benzodiazapine binding sites in audiogenic seizure-susceptible mice. *J Neurochem* 1982; 39: 864–70.

(31) Olsen RW, Wamsley JK, McCabe RT, Less RJ, Lomax P. Benzodiazapine-/gamma-aminobutyric acid receptor deficit in the midbrain of the seizure-susceptible gerbil. *Proc Natl Acad Sci USA* 1985; 82: 6701–5.

(32) Lloyd KG, Bossi L, Morselli PL, Rougier M, Loiseau P, Munari C. Biochemical evidence for dysfunction of GABA neurons in human epilepsy. In: Bartholini G, Bossi L, Lloyd KG, Morselli PL, eds. *Epilepsy and GABA receptor agonists: basic and therapeutic research*, New York: Raven Press, 1985: 43–51.

(33) Ribak CE, Harris AB, Vaughn JE, Roberts E. Inhibitory, GABAergic nerve terminals decrease at sites of focal epilepsy. *Science* 1979; 205: 211–4.

(33a) Ribak CE, Hunt CA, Bakay RAE, Oertel WH. A decrease in the number of GABAergic somata is associated with the preferential loss of GABAergic terminals at epileptic foci. *Brain Res* 1986; 363: 78–90.

(34) Ribak CE, Joubran C, Kesslak JP, Bakay RAE. A selective decrease in the number of GABAergic somata occurs in pre-seizing monkeys with alumina gel granuloma. *Epilepsy Res* 1989; 4: 126–38.

(35) Babb TL, Pretorius JK, Kupfer WR, Crandall PH. Glutamate decarboxylase-immunoreactive neurons are preserved in human epileptic hippocampus. *J Neurosci* 1989; 9: 2562–74.

(36) Ayala GF, Matsumoto H, Gumnit RJ. Excitability changes and inhibitory mechanisms in neocortical neurons during seizures. *J Neurophysiol* 1970; 33: 73–85.

(37) Herrling PL, Morris R, Salt TE. Effects of excitatory amino acids and their antagonists on membrane and action potentials of cat caudate neurones. *J Physiol* 1933; 339: 207–22.

(38) Croucher MJ, Collins JF, Meldrum BS. Anticonvulsant action of excitatory amino acids antagonists. *Science* 1982; 216: 899–901.

(39) Chapman AG. Excitatory amino acid antagonists and therapy of epilepsy. In: Meldrum BS, ed. *Excitatory amino antagonists*, Oxford: Blackwell Scientific Publications Ltd, 265–86.

(40) Geddes JW, Cahan LD, Cooper SM, Kim RC, Choi BH, Cotman CW. Altered distribution of excitatory amino acid receptors in temporal lobe epilepsy. *Exp Neurol* 1990; 108: 214–20.

(41) McDonald JW, Garofalo EA, Hood T, et al. Altered excitatory and inhibitory amino acid receptor binding in hippocampus of patients with temporal lobe epilepsy. *Ann Neurol* 1990; 29: 529–41.

(42) Louvel J, Pumain R. *N*-Methyl-D aspartate-mediated response in epileptic cortex in man: an in vitro study. In: Engel J, ed., *Neurotransmitters, seizures and epilepsy IV*, New York: Demos Publishers 1991: 487–95.

(43) Mody I, Stanton PK, Heinemann U. Activation of *N*-methyl-D-aspartate receptors parallels changes in cellular and synaptic properties of dentate granule cells after kindling. *J Neurophysiol* 1988; 59: 1033–53.

(44) Nadler JV, Perry BW, Cotman CW. Selective reinnervation of hippocampal area CA1 and the fascia dentata after destruction of CA3-AC4 afferents with kainic acid. *Brain Res* 1980; 182: 1–9.

(45) Steriade M, Llinas RR. The functional states of the thalamus and the associated neuronal interplay. *Physiol Rev* 1988; 68: 649–742.

(46) Coulter DA, Huguenard JR, Prince DA. Differential effects of petit mal anticonvulsants and convulsants on thalamic neurones: GABA current blockade. *Brit J Pharmacol* 1990; 100: 807–13.

(47) Neumann PE, Seyfried TN. Mapping of two genes that influence susceptibility to audiogenic seizures in crosses of C57BL/6J and DBA/2J mice. *Behav Genet* 1990; 20: 307–23.

(48) Shin C, McNamara JO, Morgan JI, Curran T, Cohen DR. Induction of c-fos mRNA expression by afterdischarge in the hippocampus of naive and kindled rats. *J Neurochem* 1990; 55: 1050–5.

(49) Gall CM, Isackson PJ. Limbic seizures increase neuronal production of messenger RNA for nerve growth factor. *Science* 1989; 245: 758–61.

New developments in neuroimaging in schizophrenia

L S PILOWSKY AND R KERWIN

Introduction

Neuroimaging techniques developed for elucidating brain structure and function provide neuropsychiatry with a powerful investigatory tool. There are now a plethora of studies examining brain structure and function in schizophrenia using neuropathological and neuroimaging approaches.

The neuropathology of schizophrenia is addressed by Roberts (Chapter 2). This review will focus on neuroimaging approaches to research in schizophrenia; structural (computerized tomography (CT) and magnetic resonance imaging (MRI)) and functional (positron emission tomography (PET) and single photon emission tomography (SPET)).

Neuroimaging provides an opportunity to reassess post-mortem findings in the living human brain, controlling for the effects of treatment, in representative groups of patients matched closely with controls and allowing correlations to be made with clinical or neuropsychological variables in life.

Structural imaging

Pneumoencephalographic studies were the first to provide structural imaging data in schizophrenia. They revealed ventricular enlargement in schizophrenic patients[1,2,3]. Follow-up after 20 years showed this enlargement to be static, or nonprogressive[4]. These changes were related to the clinical defect state of personality disintegration and poor outcome.

The major advance in structural imaging came with the development of noninvasive techniques using computerized methods to construct 3-dimensional images from 2-dimensional data[5].

Computerized tomography (CT) has been applied extensively to schizophrenia research. Lewis[6] has reviewed the area comprehensively. This article will provide only a brief introduction to structural imaging. Lewis[6]

All correspondence to: Dr LS Pilowsky, Institute of Psychiatry, De Crespigny Park, Denmark Hill, London SE5 8AF.

Cambridge Medical Reviews: Neurobiology and Psychiatry Volume 1 highlighted the following methodological considerations which may lead to artefact: patient selection, choice of controls, methods of measurement and criteria distinguishing normal from abnormal. These considerations apply to all methods of neuroimaging and so will be discussed in some detail.

Operational criteria for psychiatric disorder have ensured reasonable standardization of diagnosis. Patients may still differ in important ways; such as demographic, clinical and in the treatments they are receiving. Lewis[6] suggests that efforts should be directed at using epidemiologically consistent samples, such as consecutive admissions from a defined catchment area. Exclusion criteria also vary; the most common are: preexisting neurological disease, mental impairment, upper age limit and concurrent physical illness. Other studies have barred heavy alcohol consumers, females, abnormalities on EEG and L handers.

Controls must also be selected carefully, with the same criteria used for patients applied to them. Factors influencing brain structure have included social class[7], weight, ethnicity[8] and educational level[9].

Variations may also occur between researchers in interpretation of imaging data. For example, Andreasen[10] pointed out that differences between groups in defining cut-off points for ventricular enlargement could account for conflicting findings.

Measurement of brain regions is sometimes performed visually (leading to problems in identifying the fluid/brain edge). In CT this has been replaced largely by automated techniques using the original CT data, thus improving reliability. In all image analysis techniques, the attempt is made to attain high levels of interpreter reliability and rating of data blind to patient or control status.

CT scan findings and schizophrenia

CT studies substantiated the earlier findings of pneumoencephalography. Johnstone et al[11] and others[12,13] demonstrated ventriculomegaly in schizophrenic patients. Other studies show structural changes to be present at the onset of positive symptoms[13,14] and in some cases before florid illness emerges[15]. The changes, like those found by pneumoencephalographic studies were shown to be nonprogressive[16,17]. In a review of 21 studies using prospectively ascertained healthy controls scanned concurrently with the patient group Lewis[6] concluded that there was consistent evidence of relative enlargement of the third and lateral ventricles and cortical sulci in some patients.

The specificity of the changes to schizophrenia is as yet uncertain. Harvey et al[18], in a series of consecutively admitted patients with functional psychoses and matched community controls did not find diagnostic specificity for increased ventricular brain ratio. The lateral ventricular size of bipolar patients lay between that of schizophrenics and controls.

Researchers have attempted to correlate CT changes with a variety of clinical indices. Increases in ventricular brain ratio have been associated with evidence of premorbid psychopathology[19]. Many, but not all studies report a relationship with neuropsychological impairment[11,20,21]. Johnstone et al[22] demonstrated that cognitive impairment was significantly related to brain area in early onset, but not in late onset cases. Murray et al[23] noted that the former group of patients are far more likely to be male and to have shown personality and cognitive deficits in childhood[24,25]. Erel et al[26] examined the relationship between ventricular enlargement and prospectively assessed deficits in premorbid school/occupational adjustment in 34 subjects on the Copenhagen schizophrenia high-risk register. Ventricular enlargement was significantly correlated with poor premorbid adjustment irrespective of diagnosis. Weinberger[19] correlated increased ventricular size with poor response to treatment, but this finding in itself does not consistently predict response to antipsychotic medication[27].

MRI and schizophrenia
MRI, has emerged as the main research tool in structural imaging. MRI generates images based on radiofrequency signals emitted by hydrogen nuclides when excited by radiofrequency pulses. Several components of the signal are used: the proton density, the spin-lattice relaxation time (T_1) and the spin–spin relaxation time (T_2). These indices vary in different tissues and in pathology. Besson[28] suggests that relaxation times tend to increase in most pathological conditions. In the brain relaxation time is greatest in the CSF followed by grey matter then white matter in decreasing order. MRI is safer in that it does not employ ionizing radiation, has higher resolution and is better able to distinguish grey from white matter structures[29].

Studies performed so far using MRI have also shown smaller volume of brain structures in schizophrenia, particularly the temporal lobe and the hippocampus[22,30-34]. Bogerts et al[32] noted that hippocampal volume was significantly smaller in the left hemisphere of male patients. Nasrallah et al[35] noted an overall decrease in cerebral volume in schizophrenics. Harvey et al[36] studied 48 schizophrenics and 34 healthy controls. They also found a significant decrease in cerebral volume in schizophrenics (due to a selective decrease in cortical volume with a corresponding increase in sulcal fluid volume). They did not detect a particular loss of volume in the hippocampal/amygdala complex, but noted a reversal of the normal pattern of asymmetry in schizophrenics.

Others have attempted to match clinical or neuropsychological findings with structural abnormalities. Persaud et al[37] found a significant inverse correlation between basal ganglia volume size and negative symptoms in schizophrenics. Young et al[38] also correlated severity of negative symptoms with bilateral reduction in size of head of caudate. Raine et al[39] reported that schizophrenics' poor performance on the Wisconsin Card Sorting test was correlated with a bilateral decrease in frontal lobe volume.

MRI has been applied to twin populations, attempting to disentangle the role of acquired or genetic factors. Suddath[31] studied 15 pairs of monozygotic twins discordant for schizophrenia. Findings in affected twins included: increased ventricular size (particularly in the lateral and third ventricle), and bilateral loss of hippocampal volume.

Further MRI studies will undoubtedly attempt to refine these preliminary clinical, neuropsychological and morphological correlations. An emerging application of MRI is in the field of magnetic resonance spectroscopy, a technique which allows the calculation of concentrations of endogenous substances in body tissues.

Functional imaging

Advances in imaging technology over the last decade, have permitted examination of brain function in the living human. Now it is possible to measure cerebral metabolism and blood flow, neurotransmitters and neurotransmitter receptor populations in vivo. Imaging with both PET and SPET is based on regional localization and quantification within tissue of compounds labelled with either positron (PET) or gamma emitting radioisotopes (SPET). Maurer[40] has compared PET and SPET imaging. PET confers advantages in terms of sensitivity and resolution (and this is consistently increasing), but is extremely expensive. This is because an on-site cyclotron is needed to manufacture positron emitting isotopes. Thus only a few centres are able to afford the technology and expertise required. More recently, SPET has begun to rise to the challenge set by PET imaging, with great improvements in sensitivity and resolution. In addition, the development of ligands for SPET which may be radiolabelled without loss of biological activity has increased its potential as a research tool. Because SPET has much lower running costs than PET, it is possible to investigate much larger samples, such that earlier PET findings in schizophrenia may be substantiated and extended by SPET imaging.

Hypotheses relating to brain function may be tested in the resting state and in response to psychomotor or pharmacological challenges. Differences in response may then be compared across a variety of physiological and pathophysiological conditions. Clearly, rigorous methodology is needed in functional studies as state-dependent variables are measured. Thus, subjects should be characterized in terms of diagnosis, physical and demographic detail, and mental/physical symptoms at the time of scanning. The subjects physiological state during the scan is important, factors such as eyes open or closed, light levels or noise in the room, will need to be taken into account. Also of importance is the subject's state of emotional arousal, or thinking patterns, particularly in psychological activation tasks.

Data acquired from PET studies are incorporated into mathematical models which describe the biological processes under examination, such that the parameter of interest can be derived[41]. With regard to cerebral tissue metabolism, PET measures rates of metabolism either by the rate of utilization of a substrate (the oxygen technique) or the accumulation of a product (the deoxyglucose technique). Crucial to interpretation of the results in brain tissue is the fact that cerebral activity is almost entirely dependent on oxidative metabolism, using oxygen and glucose as substrates[42]. SPET techniques have focused on the measurement of cerebral blood flow, initially using radioisotopes of inert gases (^{133}Xe) but now employing lipid soluble radiotracers (for example ^{99}Tc^{m} HMPAO) which cross the blood–brain barrier freely and, due to an intracellular pH change become trapped inside the cell[43]. The resulting image gives a 'freeze frame' of cerebral blood flow at the time of the scan. Most early blood flow studies used the inert gas method and so were unable to localize cerebral blood flow with SPET to the extent that is possible today.

PET and SPECT measures of cerebral metabolism and blood flow in schizophrenia

Frackowiack et al[44] found cerebral metabolism and perfusion to be tightly coupled. In the following discussion findings in each are not separated. The earliest study of global cerebral blood flow (CBF) using the nitrous oxide method failed to report differences between normals and schizophrenics (Kety and Schmidt[45]). Later, Ingvar and Franzen[46] using inhaled ^{133}xenon found a relative decrease in rCBF in the frontal cortex of schizophrenics. A method for measuring cerebral metabolism emerged with the development of ^{18}FDG PET. ^{18}FDG is incorporated into the cell and phosphorylated but is not metabolized further by the glycolytic pathway and thus is trapped in the cell during the scanning period. It therefore is thought to reflect brain glucose uptake/demand[47]. The earlier ^{133}xenon findings were supported by Buchsbaum et al[48], in which a small series of patients showed decreased fronto-occipital ratios of glucose metabolism as measured by ^{18}FDG and PET. These results were replicated in a further study by the same group[49]. Reviewing 17 PET studies of metabolism Buchsbaum[50] noted that 12 revealed either significant or nonsignificant (or not tested) decreases in frontal–occipital ratios. When the frontal to whole brain slice ratio was used instead of the fronto-occipital ratio, hypofrontality was noted in 9 out of 10 studies reviewed. It appears that there is consistency in the studies in that decreased ^{18}FDG PET measured glucose metabolism in the frontal region is a real finding in some patients.

These studies, using small samples are at increased risk of type II errors. However, the PET glucose metabolism data is substantiated by studies examining cerebral perfusion using ^{133}xenon gamma camera methods, SPET and PET[51-54]. None the less, as Bench et al[42] point out, the notion that entire frontal lobes change as a unit in schizophrenia does not fit with current knowledge of frontal lobe neuroanatomy or physiology, and indeed current work suggests that particular regions are affected in the pre frontal cortices.

Abnormalities in cerebral metabolism and blood flow have been found in other sites. Gur et al[55] noted a higher rCBF in the left hemisphere in 19 unmedicated schizophrenics compared to 19 matched controls in the resting state. Early et al[56] reported increased cerebral blood flow to the left globus pallidus and postulated on the basis of this, and other evidence (eye tracking abnormalities in schizophrenics, relative right hemineglect, experiments in lesioned rodents) a model of schizophrenia based on a unilateral dopaminergic deficit on the right side. Buchsbaum et al's[52] finding of a relative decrease in PET measured cerebral glucose metabolism on the right side is not inconsistent with the blood flow research. Functional activity in the temporal region has not been fully examined as yet. Post-mortem and structural imaging research would indicate abnormalities in this region. Initial studies have shown decreases in metabolism and perfusion in the temporal region compared to normal controls[49, 53, 57]. Future studies should improve data acquisition methods to specifically examine this region.

Researchers have also attempted to correlate clinical state with PET and SPET data. Warkentin et al[54] studied rCBF repeatedly during a psychotic episode in 17 patients; 7 medicated and 10 medication free. The [133]xenon inhalation method was used. They found that patients with a clinical exacerbation of their condition had normal blood flow, but that this redistributed during remission to produce low flow in frontal areas. The anteroposterior ratios correlated with the degree of behavioural disturbance. Wolkin et al[53] using [18]FDG PET also showed persistence of hypofrontality in a group of 10 chronic schizophrenic subjects before and after neuroleptic treatment. Other areas which had been hypoactive (temporal) or hyperactive (basal ganglia) returned to normal levels following treatment. These findings were supported by those of DeLisi et al[58] in a PET study of chronically treated patients off and on medication. Kishimoto et al[59] distinguished a 'hypofrontal' group of schizophrenic patients with flat, blunted affect and a 'hypoparietal' group with delusions and hallucinations.

Examining the effects of acute antipsychotic administration (single dose of intravenous thiothixene) on regional brain metabolism in four never medicated chronic schizophrenics vs twelve controls, Volkow et al[60] did not find a significant effect of neuroleptic or evidence of hypofrontality. On the basis of this study they suggest that hypofrontality may be secondary to chronic neuroleptic treatment. A persistent increase in basal ganglia activity was noted, on and off medication.

It appears then that deranged cerebral metabolism and blood flow is present in schizophrenia. Garza-Trevino et al[29] identify two subgroups, one chronically ill with more negative symptoms, showing decreased frontal metabolism, another, with a shorter duration of illness and no impairment in frontal activity. Both subgroups show increases in basal ganglia activity. Other research has attempted to carefully define patients clinically and neuro-psychologically prior to scanning. Liddle et al[61] studied 26 patients with DSM III chronic schizophrenia during the stable phase of their illness. They divided patients into the following subsyndromes depending on the dominant symptomatology. These were: psychomotor poverty, disorganization, and reality distortion syndromes. Using the ^{15}O inhalation technique, patients cerebral blood flow was compared to that of controls at rest.

Of particular interest to investigators looking at dynamic indices such as cerebral perfusion and metabolism, are pattern alterations deviating from the normal in response to a variety of challenges. An early example of this is the study of Weinberger et al[62]. They used the ^{133}xenon inhalation method to determine rCBF in 20 medication free schizophrenics and 25 normal controls. Two tests were administered during scanning. These were the Wisconsin Card Sort (WCST) (specific for the dorsolateral prefrontal cortex (DLPFC)) and a simple number matching test. Flow to the DLPFC was clearly increased during the WCST in controls but not patients (the number matching did not affect flow to this area in patients or controls). The results were replicated in further sample of neuroleptic treated patients vs controls (Berman et al[63]). The degree to which blood flow to the DLPFC was increased correlated with performance on the WCST.

This approach, correlating performance on a neuropsychological task designed to elicit a response from a specific brain region paves the way for studies which enhance understanding, not only of deficits in schizophrenia or other neuropsychiatric syndromes, but of normal psychophysiology.

PET and SPET and receptor measurement

PET and SPET techniques allow for estimation of receptor density and activity in vivo. Now, a variety of receptor systems may be studied quantitatively at different stages in the evolution of the disease process. In schizophrenia research, the dopaminergic system has received greatest attention. A linear correlation has been demonstrated between antipsychotic drug affinity for the dopamine D2 receptor in animal brains in vitro and clinical antipsychotic potency in man[64]. No other receptor system so far studied has shown such a direct correlation for schizophrenia. This, and other evidence underpinning the dopamine hypothesis of schizophrenia, suggests that, in schizophrenia, there is an apparent overactivity of dopaminergic mechanisms in crucial brain regions.

A variety of ligands have been developed for use in PET and SPET experiments. These have in common: high affinity for the D2 receptor in vivo with saturable and specific binding, low non-specific binding, capacity to pass through the blood/brain barrier easily, retention of these characteristics even when radiolabelled, metabolites which do not interfere with binding in the site under investigation and rapid clearance of the tracer from the blood. One of the first ligands, ^{11}C-N-methylspiperone (NMSP) has high affinity for D2 receptors, but also binds appreciably to 5HT2 receptors. Now, there are other more specific ligands, for example: the substituted benzamides (e.g.: raclopride (PET), IBZM (SPET)) and ergolines (bromolisuride-PET). When radiolabelled they should be of high specific activity and are given in minute amounts, such that they do not participate in the mass action of the endogenous agent at the receptor site under investigation[65].

The neostriatum is the site chosen for examination of D2 receptors in PET and SPET research. This site is rich in D2 receptors and the large number of receptors permits precise quantification with currently available methods[66]. There is evidence that there may be abnormalities in the basal ganglia in schizophrenia[56,57], and that patients with basal ganglia disease such as Huntington's or Parkinson's have some symptoms in common with schizophrenic patients. In addition, the nucleus accumbens, closely connected with the limbic system where abnormalities have been proposed, is contiguous with the basal ganglia in humans.

The striatum to cerebellar ratio is taken as the index of specific D2 receptor binding. The model is based on the accumulation of the radiolabelled ligand in the striatum, while a region devoid of receptors represents an approximation to nonspecific binding (cerebellum). Over time the ratio increases, the rate of increase giving an index of ligand binding (this rate of increase also depends on cerebral perfusion to the region under examination)[67]. A different model involves comparison of two measurements of D2 receptors using NMSP PET, one with and one without haloperidol. Receptor density is estimated by comparing the difference in NMSP concentrations in scans obtained in the blocked and unblocked states[29].

The earliest study assessing D2 receptor status in vivo employed [77]Br bromospiperone and gamma camera technology[68]. An 11% increase of the striatum:cerebellum ratio was reported in patients, many of whom had been neuroleptic treated. PET studies in never treated schizophrenics initially gave conflicting results. A group from Johns Hopkins[69] using ^{11}C NMSP reported striking elevations in Bmax (D2 receptor density) in 10 antipsychotic drug naive and 5 previously treated schizophrenic patients compared to 11 normal controls. A study from the Karolinska group[70,71] using ^{11}C raclopride and an equilibrium model compared 20 healthy subjects and 18 drug naive schizophrenic patients. They found no differences between schizophrenics and controls in Bmax or Kd(affinity). A workshop was convened to fully examine these discrepancies[66]. It was felt that several factors could have contributed to the divergencies, including; patient and control characteristics, differences in brain regions examined, inter-ligand differences (specificity of binding, metabolism, clearance from the blood) different mathematical models, variability in PET instrumentation techniques and other factors. These in themselves were not thought to account for the different findings but may have had a cumulative effect. The workshop concluded that more attention to definition of patient and control characteristics was indicated as well as more basic research into the kinetics of radioligand behaviour to establish the most appropriate kinetic model.

Since then, a further group has published data comparing 9 drug naive and 3 drug-free schizophrenic patients with 12 controls[72]. Using the equilibrium method and [76]Br bromospiperone PET, no differences were found between patients and controls. A follow-up study by the same group[73], this time using [76]Br-bromolisuride in 10 drug naive and 9 drug free patients compared to 14 normal controls was also negative. Thus, the results so far would suggest no quantitative difference between striatal D2 dopamine receptors in schizophrenic patients and controls when the patients are taken as a homogeneous group.

Although no major global differences have been noted, some intriguing findings have been reported. For example, Farde et al[71] found significantly higher densities in the left than in the right putamen (but not the caudate nucleus) in schizophrenic patients but not controls. This fits with the work showing increased perfusion and metabolism in the basal ganglia on the left side[56,57]. Martinot et al[73] noted that subchronic patients had higher ratios than chronically ill patients whereas Wong et al found increased D2 density in chronic patients. In the more recent study by Martinot et al, this finding was not replicated. None the less, state dependent variables could account for differences within patient samples and will have to be elucidated in the future.

Another application of this technique is in the field of pharmacology. Farde et al[74] using ^{11}C raclopride PET determined central D2 receptor occupancy in the putamen of schizophrenic patients treated with 11 chemically distinct antipsychotic drugs. They found that clinical treatment of patients with these drugs resulted in a 65–85% occupancy of the receptor by the drug. This provided the first support in the living human for the notion that the degree of D2 receptor blockade is responsible for the mechanism of action of antipsychotics. No occupancy of striatal D2 receptors was demonstrated in a patient on nortryptiline. The blockade of D2 receptors was dose dependent and reversible. Following withdrawal of medication a curvilinear relationship was demonstrated between central D2 occupancy and serum drug concentrations. Farde et al[75] using the selective D1 receptor ligand SCH23390 and PET demonstrated that, of all the antipsychotics, only clozapine blocked D1 receptors to nearly the same extent as it blocked D2 receptors. Others have proposed studying receptor systems and cerebral metabolism in response to pharmacological activation by agonists or antagonists[65]. This research pro-

L S Pilowsky & R Kerwin

vides exciting opportunities to test hypotheses relating to antipsychotic pharmacodynamics and clinical response in the living human, as well as answering basic neurochemical questions relating to schizophrenia.

Conclusion

This chapter has sketched a brief introduction into recent work in the field of neuroimaging and schizophrenia. The area is constantly changing, with increasingly sophisticated instrumentation, research paradigms, mathematical modelling and data analysis. The work discussed here will be re-evaluated in the light of new findings.

References

(1) Jacobi W, Winkler H. Encephalographische Studien an chronisch Schizophrenen. *Arch Psychiatr Nervenkr* 1927; 81: 299–332.
(2) Lempke R. Unntersuchungen über die soziale Prognose der Schizophrenic unter besonderer Berücksichtigung des encephalographischen Befundes. *Arch Psychiatri Nervenkr* 1935; 104: 89–136.
(3) Huber G. Pneumoencephalographische and psychopathologische Bilder bei endogen Psychosen. Berlin: Springer-Verlag, 1957.
(4) Huber G, Gross G, Schutter R. A long term follow-up study of schizophrenia: psychiatric course of illness and prognosis. *Acta Psychiatr Scan* 1975; 52: 49–57.
(5) Abou-Saleh MT. Brain imaging in psychiatry [Editorial preface]. *Br J Psychiat* 1990; 157 (suppl 9): 7–10.
(6) Lewis S. Computerised tomography in schizophrenia 15 years on. *Br J Psychiat* 1990; 157 (suppl 9): 16–25.
(7) Pearlson GD, Garbacz DJ, Moberg PJ et al. Symptomatic, familial, perinatal and social correlates of computerized axial tomography (CAT) changes in schizophrenics and bipolars. *J Nerv Ment Dis* 1985; 173: 42–50.
(8) Nimgaonkar V, Wessley S, Murray RM. Prevalence of familiality, obstetric complications and structural brain damage in schizophrenic patients. *Br J Psychiat* 1988; 153: 191–7.
(9) DeMyer MK, Gilmar RL, Hendrie HC et al. Magnetic resonance brain images in schizophrenic and normal subjects: influence of diagnosis and education. *Schizophrenia Bull* 1988; 14: 21–38.
(10) Andreasen NC, Smith MR, Jacoby CG, Dennert JW, Oken SA. Ventricular enlargement in schizophrenia, definition and prevalence. *Am J Psychiat* 1982; 139: 292–6.
(11) Johnstone EC, Crow TJ, Frith CD, Husband J, Kreel L. Cerebral ventricular size and cognitive impairment in chronic schizophrenia. *Lancet* 1976; ii: 924–6.
(12) Nasrallah HA, Jacoby CG, McCalley-Whitters M, Kuperman S. Cerebral ventricular enlargment in subtypes of chronic schizophrenia. *Arch Gen Psychiat* 1982; 39: 774–7.
(13) Turner SW, Toone BK, Brett-Jones JR. Computerised tomographic scan changes in early schizophrenia. Preliminary findings. *Psych Med* 1986; 16: 219–25.
(14) Schulz SC, Koller MM, Kishore PR, Hamer RM, Gehl JJ, Friedel RO. Ven-

tricular enlargement in teenage patients with schizophrenia spectrum disorder. *Am J Psychiat* 1983: 1592–5.

(15) O'Callaghan E, Larkin C, Redmond O, Stack J, Ennis JT, Waddington JL. Early onset schizophrenia after teenage head injury. *Br J Psychiat* 1988; 153: 394–6.

(16) Illowsky B, Juliano DM, Bigelow LB, Weinberger DR. Stability of CT scan findings in schizophrenia. *J Neurol Neurosurg Psychiat* 1988; 51: 209–13.

(17) Vita A, Sacchetti I, Valvassoni G, Cazullo CL. Brain morphology in schizophrenia: a 20 year CT scan follow-up study. *Acta Psychiat Scand* 1988; 78: 618–21.

(18) Harvey I, Williams M, Toone BK, Lewis SW, Turner SW, McGuffin P. The ventricular-brain ratio (VBR) in functional psychoses: the relationship of lateral ventricular and total intracranial area. *Psych Med* 1990; 20: 55–62.

(19) Weinberger DR, Cannon-Spoor E, Potkin SG, Wyatt RJ. Poor premorbid adjustment and CT scan abnormalities in chronic schizophrenia. *Am J Psychiat* 1980; 137: 1410–13.

(20) Crow TJ. The two syndrome concept: origins and current status. *Schizophrenia Bull* 1985; 11: 471–585.

(21) Golden CJ, Moses JA, Zelazowski R, Graber B et al. Cerebral ventricular size and neuropsychological impairment in young chronic schizophrenics. *Arch Gen Psychiat* 1980; 37: 619–23.

(22a) Johnstone EC, Owens DGC, Bydder GM, Colter N, Crow TJ, Frith CD. The spectrum of structural brain changes in schizophrenia: age of onset as a predictor of cognitive and clinical impairments and their cerebral correlates. *Psych Med* 1989; 19: 91–103.

(22b) Johnstone EC, Owens DGC, Crow TJ et al. Temporal lobe structure as determined by nuclear magnetic resonance in schizophrenia and bipolar affective disorder. *J Neurol Neurosurg Psychiat* 1989; 52: 736–41.

(23) Murray RM, Jones P, O'Callaghan E. Foetal brain development and later schizophrenia. *Proceedings of Ciba Symposium No. 156: The childhood environment and adult disease.* 1990: in press.

(24) Aylward E, Walker E, Bettes B. Intelligence in schizophrenia: meta-analysis of the research. *Schizophrenia Bull* 1984; 10: 430–59.

(25) Foerster A, Lewis S, Owen M, Murray RM. Do risk factors for schizophrenia also predict poor premorbid functioning in psychosis? *Schizophrenia Res* 1990; in press.

(26) Erel O, Cannon TD, Meggin-Hollister J et al. Ventricular enlargement and premorbid deficits in school – occupational attainment in a high risk sample. *Schizophrenia Res* 1991; 4: 49–52.

(27) Nimgaonkar VL, Wessely S, Tune LE, Murray RM. Response to drugs in schizophrenia, the influence of family history, obstetric complications and ventricular enlargement. *Psychol Med* 1988; 18: 583–92.

(28) Besson JAO. Magnetic resonance imaging and its applications in neuropsychiatry. *Br J Psychiat* 1990; 157 (suppl 9): 25–38.

(29) Garza-Trevino E, Volkow ND et al. Neurobiology of schizophrenic syndromes. *Hosp Commun Psychiat* 1990; 41: 971–80.

(30) Suddath RL, Casanova MF, Goldberg TE, Daniel DG, Kelsae JR, Weinberger

DR. Temporal lobe pathology in schizophrenia: a quantitative magnetic resonance imaging study. *Am J Psychiat* 1989; 146: 464–72.

(31) Suddath RI, Christison GW, Torrey EF. Anatomical abnormalities in the brains of monozygotic twins discordant for schizophrenia. *N Eng J Med* 1990; 322: 789–94.

(32) Bogerts B, Ashtari M, De Greef G et al. Reduced temporal limbic structure volumes on magnetic resonance images in first episode schizophrenia. *Psychiat Res neuroimaging* 1990; 35: 1–13.

(33) Andreasen NC, Nasrallah HA, Dunn V et al. Structural abnormalities in the frontal system in schizophrenia. A magnetic resonance imaging study. *Arch Gen Psychiat* 1986; 43: 136–44.

(34) De Lisi LE et al. Perinatal complications and reduced size of brain limbic structures in familial schizophrenia. *Schizophrenia Bull* 1988; 14: 185–91.

(35) Nasrallah HA, Caffman JA, Schwarzkopf SB, Olson SL. Reduced cerebral volume in schizophrenia. *Schizophrenia Res* 1990; 3: 17.

(36) Harvey I, Ron MA, du Boulay G, Wicks D, Lewis SW, Murray RM. Diffuse reduction of cortical volume in schizophrenia on magnetic resonance imaging. *Psych Med* 1991; in press.

(37) Persaud RD, Pearlson GD, Aylward EH et al. Relationship of basal ganglia volumes to negative symptoms in schizophrenia – a magnetic resonance imaging investigation, 1991; unpublished data.

(38) Young AH, Blackwood DHR, Roxborough H, McQueen JK et al. A magnetic resonance imaging study of schizophrenia: Brain structure and clinical symptoms. *Br J Psychiat* 1991; 158: 158–64.

(39) Raine A, Reynolds G, Harrison G et al. Reduced frontal area and poorer frontal functioning in schizophrenic: an MRI, neuropsychological and psychophysiological examination. *Schizophrenia Res* 1990; 3: 21.

(40) Maurer AH. Nuclear medicine, PET comparisons to SPECT. *Radiol Clin N Am* 1988; 26: 1059–74.

(41) Phelps ME, Mazziotta JC, Schelberg H. *Positron emission tomography and autoradiography: principles and applications for the brain and heart.* New York: Raven Press, 1986.

(42) Bench CJ, Dolan RJ, Friston KJ, Frackowiack RSJ. Positron emission tomography in the study of brain metabolism in psychiatric and neuropsychiatric disorders. *Br J Psychiat* 1990; 157 (suppl 9): 82–96.

(43) Costa DC. Single photon emission tomography (SPET) with 99Tc^m-hexamethylpropyleamineoxime (HMPAO) in research and clinical practice – a useful tool. *Vasc Med Rev* 1990; 1: 179–201.

(44) Frackowiak RSJ, Pozzilli C, Legg NJ et al. Regional cerebral oxygen supply and utilization in dementia. *Brain* 1981; 104: 753–78.

(45) Kety SS, Schmidt C. The nitrous oxide method for quantitative determination of cerebral blood flow in man: theory, procedure and normal values. *J Clin Invest* 1998; 27: 476–83.

(46) Ingvar DH, Franzen G. Abnormalities of cerebral blood distribution in patients with chronic schizophrenia. *Acta Psychiat Scand* 1974; 50: 425–62.

(47) Pfefferbaum A, Zipursky RB. Neuroimaging studies of schizophrenia. *Schizophrenia Res* 1991; 4: 193–208.

(48) Buchsbaum MS, Ingvar DH, Kessler R et al. Cerebral glucography with positron emission tomography. *Arch Gen Psychiat* 1982; 39: 251-9.

(49) Buchsbaum MS, Nuechterlein KH, Haeir RJ et al. Glucose metabolic rate in normals and schizophrenics during the continuous performance test assessed by positron emission tomography. *Br J Psychiat* 1990; 156: 216-27.

(50) Buchsbaum MS. The frontal lobes, basal ganglia, and temporal lobes as sites for schizophrenia. *Schizophrenia Bull* 1990; 16: 379-89.

(51) Vita A, Cazullo CL, Invernizzi G. Cerebral SPECT in drug free schizophrenic patients, *Schizophrenia Res* 1990; 3: 24.

(52) Buchsbaum MS, Haeir RJ. Functional and anatomical brain imaging: impact on schizophrenia research. *Schizophrenia Bull* 1987; 13: 115-32.

(53) Wolkin A, Jaeger J, Brodie JD, et al. Persistence of cerebral metabolic abnormalities in chronic schizophrenia as determined by positron emission tomography. *Am J Psychiat* 1985; 142: 564-71.

(54) Warkentin S, Nilsson A, Risberg J et al. Regional cerebral blood flow in schizophrenia: repeated studies during a psychotic episode. *Psychiat Res: neuroimaging* 1990; 35: 27-38.

(55) Gur RE et al. Brain function in psychiatric disorders III regional cerebral blood flow in unmedicated schizophrenics. *Arch Gen Psychiat* 1985; 42: 329-34.

(56) Early TS, Reiman EM, Raichle ME et al. Left globus pallidus abnormality in never medicated patients with schizophrenia. *Proc Natl Acad Sci USA* 1987; 84: 561-3.

(57) Gur RE, Resnick SM, Alavi A et al. Regional brain function in schizophrenia. Positron emission tomography study. *Arch Gen Psychiat* 1987; 44: 119-25.

(58) De Lisi L, Holcomb H, Cohen R et al. Positron emission tomography in schizophrenic patients with and without neuroleptic medication. *J Cereb Blood Flow Met* 1985; 5: 206-10.

(59) Kishimoto H, Kuahara H, Ohnoss et al. Three subtypes of chronic schizophrenia identified using C-glucose positron emission tomography. *Psychiat Res* 1987; 21: 285-92.

(60) Volkow N, Brodie J, Wold A. Brain metabolism in patients with schizophrenia before and after acute neuroleptic administration. *J Neurol Neurosurg Psychiat* 1986; 49: 1199-202.

(61) Liddle PF, Friston KJ, Hirsch SR, Frackowiack RSJ. Regional cerebral metabolic activity in chronic schizophrenia. *Schizophrenia Res* 1990; 3: 23-4.

(62) Weinberger DR, Berman KF, Zec RF. Physiologic dysfunction of dorsolateral prefrontal cortex in schizophrenia I. Regional Cerebral blood flow evidence. *Arch Gen Psychiat* 1986; 43: 114-24.

(63) Berman KF, Zec RF, Weinberger DR. Physiologic dysfunction of dorsolateral prefrontal cortex in schizophrenia II role of neuroleptic treatment, attention and mental effort. *Arch Gen Psychiat* 1986; 43: 126-35.

(64) Peroutka SJ, Snyder SH. Relationship of neuroleptic drug effects at brain dopamine, serotonin, α-adrenergic and histamine receptors to clinical potency. *Am J Psychiat* 1980; 137: 1518-22.

(65) Dolan R, Bench C, Friston K. Positron emission tomography in psychopharmacology. *Int Rev Psychiat* 1990; 2: 427-39.

(66) Andreasen NC, Carson R, Diksic M et al. Workshop on schizophrenia, PET

and Dopamine D2 receptors in the human neostriatum, *Schizophrenia Bull* 1988; 14: 471–84.

(67) Wagner HN, Burns HD, Dannals RF et al. Imaging dopamine receptors in the human brain by positron tomography. *Science* 1984; 221: 1264–6.

(68) Crawley JC, Crow TJ, Johnstone EC et al. Dopamine D2 receptors in schizophrenia studied in vivo. *Lancet* 1986; ii: 224–5.

(69) Wong DF, Wagner HN, Tune LE et al. Positron emission tomography reveals elevated D2 dopamine receptors in drug-naive schizophrenics. *Science* 1986; 234: 1558–62.

(70) Farde L, Wiesel FA, Hall H et al. No D2 receptor increase in PET study of schizophrenia. *Arch Gen Psychiat* 1987; 44: 671–2.

(71) Farde L, Wiesel FA, Stone-Elander S et al. D2 dopamine receptors in neuroleptic naive schizophrenic patients. *Arch Gen Psychiat* 1990; 47: 213–19.

(72) Martinot JL, Peron-Magnan P, Huret JD et al. Striatal D2 dopaminergic receptors assessed with positron emission tomography and [76]Br Bromospiperone in untreated schizophrenic patients. *Am J Psychiat* 1990; 147: 44–50.

(73) Martinot JL, Paillere-Martinot ML, Loch C, Hardy P, Poirer MF, Mazoyer B et al. The estimated density of D2 striatal receptors in schizophrenia. A study with positron emission tomography and [76]Br-bromolisuride. *Br J Psychiat* 1991; 158: 346–51.

(74) Farde L, Weisel FA, Halldin C et al. Central D2 dopamine patients treated with antipsychotic drugs. *Arch Gen Psychiat* 1988; 45: 71–6.

(75) Farde L, Halldin C, Stone-Elander S, Sedvall G. PET analysis of human dopamine receptor subtypes using 11 C-SCH 23390 and 11C raclopride. *Psychopharmacology* 1987; 92: 278–84.

Index

Numbers in italics refer to figures

acetylcholine
  in dementing illnesses *132*
  nicotinic receptors 74
adenylate cyclase
  receptor types 79–81
  second messenger system 80
  system, in Alzheimer's disease 79–81
adrenoreceptors, in Alzheimer's disease 76
agyria/pachygyria, and epilepsy 157
AIDS dementia, and subcortical
    dementia 138
  as white matter dementia 139
Alzheimer-type dementia
  differentiation from dementias 123
  neurochemical studies 124–7; [3H]-D-
    aspartic acid binding *129*; cholinergic
    neurones, retrograde degeneration 125–
    6, 131; cholinergic system changes 124,
    131; cortical pyramidal neurone
    dysfunction 125, 127; neurofibrillary
    tangles 125, 127; neurotransmitter
    binding sites 125–6
Alzheimer-type disease, as subcortical or
    cortical dementia 123–7;
    classification 131; clinical
    correlates 131–2
Alzheimer's disease
  basal forebrain neurones, shrinkage *vs*
    loss 63–4
  beta amyloid protein in cortical
    plaques 97–106
  characteristics 138
  cognitive impairment, cholinergic deficits
    and cortical morphology 64
  cortical ChAT activity 64
  cortical neurotransmitter systems 64–5
  cortical plaques 63–4, *96*; and [3H]-D-
    aspartate 66; distribution 64–5;
    formation 66; kainate binding 71–2
  [3H]-forskolin-binding deficit 79–81
  hippocampal M2 receptors 73
  hippocampal NMDA receptor binding 70–
    1
  molecular neuropathology 95–118
  muscarinic receptors 73; and pyramidal
    cells 75; ratio to pyramidal cells 74
  neurofibrillary tangles *96*; distribution 64–
    5; kainate binding 71–2; location 65
  neurotransmitter system abnormalities 61–
    83
  phosphoinositide system 81–2
  risk factors 95
  as subcortical dementia syndrome 139–50;
    ascertainment bias 146–7; ceiling
    effects 143; cerebral blood flow and
    metabolism studies, 140–1; clinical
    presentation 139; compared with
    PSNP 150; conclusions 149–50; EEG
    studies 139–40; neuropsychological
    evidence 147–8; neuropsychological test
    battery 141–2; severity 127;
    matching 141–3; speed–accuracy trade
    off and fatigue 145–6
  transmitter replacement therapy,
    outlook 83
amino acids, in aetiology of schizophrenia
    6–8
AMPA/quisqualate receptor 7
  see also quisqualate receptors
amphetamine, increase of central dopamine
    function 3
amyloid plaques, *see* cortical plaques
APP secretase activity, beta amyloid
    deposition 102
[3H]-D-aspartate
  binding 65–6
  glutamate uptake 7
[3H]D-aspartic acid binding
  in ATD and PD *129*
  in Huntington's chorea 130

basal ganglia, homovanillic acid 5
benzodiazepine receptors, reduction 78
beta amyloid, and tau protein, related
    pathologies 115
beta amyloid deposition
  APP secretase activity 102

Index

beta amyloid deposition (*cont.*)
 hereditary cerebral hemorrhage with
  amyloidosis of Dutch type 103
 molecular explanation 103
 post-translational events 103
 proposed stages *105*
beta amyloid precursors 97
 cellular localization 100
 coding region, point mutation 103
 correlation between tissue and cellular
  distributions 99
 diffuse plaques 102–3
 extracellular beta amyloid pathology 102–3
 gene, and disease locus 103
 molecular cloning of cDNAs 97–9;
  cellular localization 97
 phosphorylation by protein kinase C 102
 physiological role 99–100
 in situ hybridization studies 99
 structure 97, *98*
beta amyloid sequence, antibodies,
 subiculum/entorhinal cortex 105
Bmax 174
[^{76}Br]-bromolisuride 175
[^{77}Br]-bromospiperone 174, 175
bradyphrenia, in Parkinson's disease 148
brain development
 genetic regulation, summary 31–3
 molecular biology 30–1
 normal 28–30
brain length, area and volume, in
 schizophrenia 16–17
brain, regions affected, grey/white matter, in
 schizophrenia 19–20
brain weight, in schizophrenia 16

C-N-methylspiperone 174
[^{11}C]-raclopride 174
Ca^{2+} conductances and epileptogenesis 161
category test, schizophrenia 45
caudate nucleus, dopamine D1 receptor 4
cerebral asymmetries, in schizophrenia 9
cerebral blood flow
 and metabolism in schizophrenia,
  imaging 171–3
 in subcortical dementias 140–1
cerebral cortex
 major afferent cholinergic projections 62
 neuronal loss 63
ChAT, *see* choline acetyltransferase

cholecystokinin (CCK)
 in Alzheimer's disease 77–8
 co-localization with tyrosine hydroxylase,
  in schizophrenia 5–6
 receptors, hippocampus 6
choline acetyltransferase (ChAT)
 loss in Alzheimer-type dementia 124–6
 loss in Alzheimer's disease 62–3
 in Parkinson's disease 127
 reduced levels in Alzheimer's disease 74
 reduction in activity, and nicotinic
  receptor loss 74
cholinergic neurones in ATD, retrograde
  degeneration 125–6
cholinergic receptors, in Alzheimer's
  disease 73–5
cholinergic system; changes in Alzheimer-
  type dementia 124; in demented and
  non-demented patients 127
 role in Alzheimer's disease 62–79;
  adrenoreceptors 76; cholinergic
  receptors 73–5; cortical interneuronal
  systems 76–9; glutamate receptors 65–
  73; role of cholinergic system 62–79;
  serotonin receptors 75–6
coagulation factor XIa, inhibition by
  protease nexin II 99
cognitive impairment, and structural changes
  in schizophrenia 22–31
computerized tomography in
  schizophrenia 167, 168–9
Continuous Performance Test (CPT),
  schizophrenia 48
corpus striatum, increased dopamine
  density 4
cortex
 alteration in schizophrenia 50–1
 number of radial units (columns) 30
cortical dementia, *see* dementias
cortical interneuronal systems, in
  Alzheimer's disease 76–9
cortical plaques
 GABAergic neurones 77
 and somatostatin-like immunoreactivity 77
cortical pyramidal neurones, loss in
  Alzheimer's disease 65
cortical receptors, somatostatin, presynaptic
  location 78–9
corticotrophin releasing factor, in
  Alzheimer's disease 77–8
cytomegalovirus, and epilepsy 157

decompression sickness, as white matter dementia 139
dementia praecox, Kraepelin 39–40
dementias, acetylcholine synthesis 64
dementias, cortical, neurochemical studies 123–35
dementias, cortical and subcortical differentiation 123–4
  neurochemical studies; classification 131; clinical correlates 131–2
dementias, multi-infarct, and Alzheimer's disease, EEC studies 139
dementias, subcortical, as clinical syndrome, definition 137–54
  cerebral blood flow and metabolism studies 140–1
  EEC studies 138–9
  neuropsychological evidence 141–9; ascertainment bias 146–7; ceiling effects 143–5; matching for severity 141–3; severity 127; speed–accuracy trade off and fatigue 145–6; with or without white matter involvement 138–9
  neurochemical studies 123–35
  see also AIDS dementia, Alzheimer's disease, Huntington's chorea, Parkinson's disease, Pick's disease, Progressive supernuclear palsy
dementias, white matter 138–9
depression, mental slowing, and subcortical dementia 138
diffuse Lewy body dementia, neurochemical studies 129
diffuse plaques, beta amyloid precursors 102–3
DLPFC, activation 47, 49
dopamine, in aetiology of schizophrenia 3–5
dopamine D1 receptor
  binding 5
  density 4–5
dopamine D2 receptor
  binding 5
  neuroleptic drugs 3–4
  PET and SPET imaging in schizophrenia 173–6; [^{11}C]-raclopride 174; [^{76}Br]-bromolisuride 175; [^{77}Br]-bromospiperone 174, 175; Bmax 174; C-N-methylspiperone 174; ligands 173–4; pharmacological approaches 175–6;

right putamen density 175; SCH 23390 175
dopamine markers
  in ATD 125, 132
  in dementing illnesses 132
dopamine-β-hydroxylase activity in ATD and PD, 128
dopamine-neuropeptide, interactions, in schizophrenia 6
dorsal raphe, serotonin 63
dorsolateral lesions, behavioral deactivation, in schizophrenia 41–3

electroencephalography, in subcortical dementias, 139–40
entorhinal cortex, cytoarchitecture, in schizophrenia 22
epilepsies(y)
  absence 155, 156, 157
  benign myoclonic in infancy 155, 156
  benign neonatal familial 155, 156
  cellular and molecular basis 155–65
  excitatory neurotransmission abnormalities 160–1
  febrile convulsions 155
  GABAergic deficits 159–60
  genetic basis 155–6
  juvenile myoclonic 155, 156, 157
  membrane conductance abnormalities 161
  mesial temporal sclerosis 158
  network abnormalities and consequences of activity 161–2
  and neuronal heterotopia 157
  neuronal migration disorders 157–8
  primary and secondary without inherited element 156, 157
  secondary 156, 157–8
  sprouting 159
excitatory amino acid neurotransmission abnormalities in epilepsy, 160–61
excitatory amino acid as transmitter for neurofibrillary tangles, ATD 125–7, 131, 132

18FDG PET in schizophrenia 171, 172
[^{3}H]-forskolin binding autoradiography 79
frontal cortex, number of large neurones 62
frontal lobe
  compromise by extra-frontal lesions 52–3
  injury, schizophrenic symptoms and behavioral changes 40–52

Index

frontal lobe (*cont.*)
  lesions, Wisconsin Card Sorting Test 44–5
  schizophrenia, structure, function, and
    connectivity 39–54

GABA
  in Alzheimer's disease 77–9
  /benzodiazepine receptor abnormalities in
    epilepsy 159
  in dementing illness *132*
  GABA A and GABA B 78
  inhibitory transmitter of cerebral cortex 6
  levels, post-mortem 3
  as transmitter in ATD, 125, *132*
GABAergic deficits in epilepsy, 159–60
GABAergic innervation, loss 77
GABAergic neurones, cortical plaques 77
gamma emitting radioisotopes (SPET) in
    schizophrenia 170–6
  cerebral metabolism and blood flow 171–3
  compared with positron emitting
    radioisotopes 170
  deoxyglucose technique 171
  incorporation of data 171
  oxygen technique 171
  and receptor measurement 173–6;
    dopamine D2 173–8
  subject's physiological state 170
gamma-aminobutyric acid, *see* GABA
gliosis, in schizophrenia, quantitative
    assessment 25–6
glutamate
  binding in prefrontal cortex 50–1
  excitatory neurotransmitter 6
  neurones, in Parkinson's disease 127
  neurons, pre- and post-synaptic
    markers 7–8
  receptors in Alzheimer's disease 65–73;
    kainate receptors 67, 68, 72–3;
    markers 65–6; NMDA receptors 67,
    69–71; quisqualate receptors 67, 68,
    72–3
  in schizophrenia, aetiology 6–8
glutamatergic receptor system, receptor sub-
    types
  AMPA/quisqualate 7
  kainic acid 7–8
  NMDA 7–8
glutamatergic terminals, [³H]-aspartate
    binding 69
Gs binding protein, adenylate cyclase 80

Hallervorden–Spatz disease, cortical Lewy
    bodies 129
hereditary cerebral hemorrhage with
    amyloidosis of Dutch type, beta amyloid
    deposition 103
HIAA, concentrations in CSF 52
Hilar interneuron, intemporal lobe
    epilepsy 159
hippocampal formation, of tau protein,
    repeat isoform transcripts, 108
hippocampal temporal sclerosis, in
    epilepsy 158
hippocampus
  CCK receptors 6
  in epilepsy: NMDA sensitivity 161;
    sprouting 159
  function and anatomy 30
  left hippocampal formation, in
    schizophrenia 20–2
  parahippocampal gyrus; anatomical
    links 29; pathology in schizophrenia 21
  pyramidal cell loss, in schizophrenia 20–1
  pyramidal cells, beta amyloid
    precursors 100–1
homovanillic acid (HVA)
  in basal ganglia 5
  concentrations in CSF 52
5-HT2, binding in prefrontal cortex 50–1
5-HT2 receptors, in Parkinson's disease 127,
    132
5-HT, *see* serotonin
Huntington's chorea
  [³H]-D-aspartic acid binding 130
  basal ganglia 130, 131
  cerebral cortex 130, 131
  differentiation from dementias 123
  as subcortical dementia syndrome 138;
    cerebral blood flow and metabolism
    studies 140; EEG studies 140;
    neuropsychological evidence 147–8;
    neuropsychological profile 142; severity
    of disease 142–6
HVA, *see* homovanillic acid
5-hydroxytryptamine, *see* serotonin

K⁺ conductances and epileptogenesis 161
kainate receptor 7–8, 67, 68, 72–73
Kraepelin, on dementia praecox 39–40

L-dopa, increase of central dopamine
    function 3

lateral ventricles, enlargement in
   schizophrenia 50
left perisylvian hypometabolism in PET
   scan, Pick's disease 149
leukoariosis, as white matter dementia 139
Lewy bodies
   in dementia 129, 123
   in subcortical dementia 149
limbic and cortical areas, dopamine
   innervation 3–4
limbic system, genesis of psychosis 43
lissencephaly, and epilepsy 157
locus coeruleus
   neurone loss 64
   noradrenaline 63

magnetic resonance imaging in
   schizophrenia 169–70
MAP2b, rat, structure 109
MAP2c, embryonic brain development 109
membrane conductance abnormalities in
   epilepsy 161
mesial temporal sclerosis, in epilepsy 158
microdysgenesis in epilepsy 157
microtubule-associated proteins MAP2 and
   MAP-U 106–8
Miller–Dieker syndrome, seizures and
   infantile spasms 157
multiple carboxylase deficiency and
   epilepsy 156
multiple sclerosis, and subcortical
   dementia 138; bradyphrenia 148–9;
   mental processing speed 148; as white
   matter dementia 139
muscarinic M1 receptors, coupling to
   associated G protein 81

N-methyl-D-aspartate (NMDA) receptor 7–
   8, 67, 69–71
   in epileptogenesis 160–1
   in schizophrenia 7–8
Na$^+$ conductances and epileptogenesis 161
neurochemical markers in ATD 125
neurofibrillary tangles
   and 5HT2 receptors 75
   in Alzheimer-type dementia 125; effect on
      severity 127
   double-labelling 114–15
   paired helical filament 106–16
   in progressive disease 123

in somatostatin-containing neurones 77
   in subcortical dementia 149
neuroleptics, increase in dopamine D2
   receptor 4
neuronal heterotopia, and epilepsy 157
neuronal migration, disorders, and
   epilepsy 157–8
neurones, numbers 62
neuropeptide Y
   in Alzheimer's disease 77–8
   markers 63
neuropeptides, aetiology of schizophrenia
   5–6
neurotensin, dopamine co-transmitter 5
neurotensin receptors, neuroleptic
   medication 6
neurotransmitter receptors, in Alzheimer's
   disease 79–81
   adenylate cyclase system 79–81
neurotransmitter system abnormalities,
   Alzheimer's disease 61–83
nicotinic receptor, loss in Alzheimer's
   disease 74
NIMH studies, twin studies 48–51
noradrenaline
   locus coeruleus 63
   loss in Parkinson's disease 127
nucleus accumbens
   dopamine D1 receptor 4
   increased dopamine density 4
nucleus basalis, neuronal loss 63

olivopontocerebellar atrophy, cortical ChAT
   activity 64

paired helical filament
   associated with tau proteins 112–13
   formation 108
   neurofibrillary tangles 106–16
   structure 106
   tau protein 106–16
parahippocampal gyrus
   asymmetric development 29–30
   function and anatomy 30
   hippocampus, anatomical links 29
   normal development 28
   projections to 31
   thinning, in schizophrenia 31
Parkinson's disease, cortical ChAT
   activity 64

Index

Parkinson's disease (*cont.*)
loss, 127; increase in muscarinic
receptors 74
neurochemical studies 127–8; [³H]-D-
aspartic acid binding 128
as subcortical or cortical dementia 123–7;
classification 131; clinical
correlates 131–2
as subcortical dementia syndrome 140–8;
ascertainment bias 146–7;
bradyphrenia 148; cerebral blood flow
and metabolism studies 140–1; EEG
studies 140; neuropsychological
evidence 147–8; severity of
disease 142–6; speed–accuracy trade off
and fatigue 145–6
Wisconsin Card Sorting Test 145
periventricular white matter disease, and
subcortical dementia 138
PET, *see* positron emitting radioisotopes
phencyclidine (PCP)
administration 7–8
receptor site 7–8
[³H]-phorbol ester binding, PKC 82
phosphoinositide system, in Alzheimer's
disease 81–2
Pick's disease
characterization 64
cortical ChAT activity 64
differentiation from dementias 123
as subcortical or cortical dementia 123;
PET scan findings 149–50; role of
ascending cholinergic system 131
PKC, [³H]-phorbol ester binding 82
plaques, *see* senile plaques
pneumoencephalographic studies in
schizophrenia 167–8
positron emitting radioisotopes in
schizophrenia 170–6
cerebral metabolism and blood flow 171–3
compared with gamma emitting
radioisotopes 170
deoxyglucose technique 171
18FDG 171
incorporation of data 171
oxygen technique 171
and receptor measurement 173; dopamine
D2, 173–5, 176
subject's physiological state 170
pre- and post-synaptic markers,
glutamate 7–8

prefrontal cortex, pathology in
schizophrenia 21
primates, non-human, 'working memory'
studies 44
progressive supranuclear palsy
striatal dopaminergic deficit 128
and subcortical dementia: cerebral blood
flow and metabolism studies 140;
definition 137; distinction from
Alzheimer's disease 138; EEG
studies 140; historical studies, 137–9;
as subcortical dementia syndrome 150;
tests, 145
protease nexin II, inhibitor of coagulation
factor XIa 99
psychosis, genesis 43
pyridoxine dependency and epilepsy 156

[³H]-quinuclidylbenzilate 73
quisqualate receptors 67, 68, 72–3

Ravens Progressive Matrices, frontal cerebral
rCBF 48
RNase protection assay, mRNAs,
location 108

SCH 23390 175
schizophrenia
aetiology: amino acids 6–8; dopamine
overactivity 3–5; neuropeptides 5–6
anatomical neuropathology 49–52
brain length, area and volume 16–17
brain weight 16
Category Test 45
cerebral asymmetries 9
children, premorbid behavioral
abnormalities 53
frontal dysfunction and cognitive
impairment 43–7
frontal lobe structure, function, and
connectivity 39–54
frontal physiological hypofunction 47–9
generalized deficit syndrome 45–7
gliosis, quantitative assessment 25–6
and glutamate, aetiology 6–8
ideational activity 41
MRI-derived measurements, consistency
with post-mortem studies 51
neuroimaging 167–80; CT scan 167, 168–
9; gamma emitting radioisotopes 170–6;
MRI 169–70; positron emitting

radioisotopes (PET) 170–6;
selection 168; structural 167–8
pathology: location 52; prefrontal –
temporolimbic connectivity 52–4
post-mortem neurochemistry 1–9
sex differences 20
structural changes: abnormal brain
development 26–8; aetiology 24–6;
laterality 23–4; normal brain
development 28–30; parahippocampal
gyrus 30
symptoms following frontal lobe
injury 40–52
temporal lobe, medial structures 19
temporal lobe pathology 15–33
ventricular system 17–18, 19
Wisconsin Card Sorting Test 44–5, 169,
173
senile dementia of Lewy body type,
neurochemical studies 129, 131, 132
senile plaques 102
in subcortical dementia 149
serotonin
dorsal raphe 63
loss in Parkinson's disease 127
serotonin markers
in ATD 125, *132*
in dementing illnesses *132*
serotonin receptors
in Alzheimer's disease 75–6
subtypes 75–6; 5HT2 receptors 75
severity of dementia, indication of type 127,
141–3
somatostatin
in Alzheimer's disease 77–8
cortical receptors, presynaptic location
78–9
in dementing illnesses *132*
markers 63
SPET, *see* gamma emitting radioisotopes
subcortical dementia, *see* dementias
subiculum, function and anatomy 30
subiculum/entorhinal cortex
antibodies, beta amyloid sequence 105
double-labelling, from Alzheimer's
disease 114
substance P, markers 63

tau antibodies, label neurofibrillary
tangles 113

tau isoforms
abnormal phosphorylation 113–14
cell protein 112
expression in *Escherichia coli* 109
tau protein
abnormally phosphorylated in Alzheimer's
disease 112–13
in Alzheimer's disease, abnormal
features 108
associated with paired helical
filaments 112–13
and beta amyloid, related pathologies 115
fetal brain, 3 repeat-containing
transcripts 108
immobilized in insoluble form 109
isoforms 107–8
and MAP2, segregation 109
mRNAs: location 108; quantitative
distribution 108
in normal brain 109
paired helical filament 106–16
recombinant, phosphorylation in vitro 112
sequence 106
transcripts, cellular localization 110
temporal limbic components, structural
abnormalities, in schizophrenia 9
temporal lobe
developmental compromise, impact on
frontal cortex 53–4
gyral pattern, schizophrenia 18–19
medial structures, in schizophrenia 19
pathology, schizophrenia 15–33
thalamic nuclei 63
tuberous sclerosis, and epilepsy 157
twin studies
anterior hippocampal size 52
monozygotic twins, generalized deficit
syndrome 46
NIMH studies 48–51
Wisconsin Card Sort 47, 49
tyrosine hydroxylase, co-localization with
CCK, in schizophrenia 5–6

vasoactive intestinal peptide, in Alzheimer's
disease 77–8
ventricular system
enlargement in schizophrenia 50
enlargement of third ventricle, in
schizophrenia 50
and reduction in hippocampal size 51
in schizophrenia 17–18, 19

Index

Wisconsin Card Sorting Test
  frontal lobe lesions 44–5
  in Parkinson's disease 145
  regional cerebral blood flow (rCBF) 47

schizophrenia 44–5, 169, 173

[133]xenon gamma in schizophrenia 171